IN THE PRESENCE OF GRIEF

IN THE PRESENCE OF GRIEF

Helping Family Members Resolve Death, Dying, and Bereavement Issues

DOROTHY S. BECVAR

Foreword by Pauline Boss

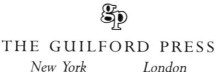

THE GUILFORD PRESS
New York   *London*

© 2001 The Guilford Press
A Division of Guilford Publications, Inc.
72 Spring Street, New York, NY 10012
www.guilford.com

Paperback edition 2003

Printed in the United States of America

This book is printed on acid-free paper.

Last digit is print number: 9 8 7 6 5 4

Library of Congress Cataloging-in-Publication Data

Becvar, Dorothy Stroh.
     In the presence of grief: helping family members resolve death,
dying, and bereavement issues / Dorothy S. Becvar; foreword by
Pauline Boss.
        p. cm.
     Includes bibliographical references and index.
     ISBN 1-57230-697-1   ISBN 1-57230-937-7
     1. Grief.   2. Bereavement—Psychological aspects.   3. Death—
Psychological aspects.   4. Loss (Psychology)   I. Title.

BF575 .G7 B435 2001
155.9'37—dc21   2001042859

The opening story in Chapter 1 is reprinted from *Death, Grief, and Caring
Relationships* (2nd ed.), by Richard Kalish. Copyright 1981 by R. A.
Kalish. Reprinted by permission of Leah McGarrigle.

The excerpt on page 262 is reprinted from *The Prophet* by Kahlil Gibran.
Copyright 1923 by Kahlil Gibran and renewed 1951 by Administrators
C.T.A. of the Kahlil Gibran Estate and Mary G. Gibran. Used by
permission of Alfred A. Knopf, a division of Random House, Inc., and
the Gibran National Committee, P. O. Box 116-5375, Bierut, Lebanon
(phone/fax: +961-1-396916; e-mail: k.gibran@cyberia.net.lb).

For all those whose stories
have enriched my story,
and especially for
Becky, Carole, Cindy, Diane, Dennis, Ingeborg,
John, Karen, Linda, Lynne, Ray, and Terry

About the Author

$\backsim$

Dorothy S. Becvar, PhD, is a licensed marital and family therapist and a licensed clinical social worker in private practice in St. Louis, Missouri. She is also president and CEO of The Haelan Centers , a not-for-profit corporation dedicated to promoting the growth and wholeness of clients in body, mind, and spirit. She has published extensively; is a well-respected teacher and trainer who has been a member of the faculties of the University of Missouri–St. Louis, St. Louis University, Texas Tech University, Washington University, and Radford University; and has presented workshops and courses both nationally and internationally on a wide variety of topics.

Foreword

∾

Death is indeed the "horse on the dining room table," the "elephant in the living room," and the one life transition everyone experiences but few want to discuss. At a time when our population is growing older, family therapists must move beyond the resistance to think and talk about death and loss. Dorothy Becvar gives us a timely gift to help.

I first read this book while sitting at my mother's bedside for what could be her last Christmas. While she slept I went to the village cemetery, trudging through deep snow to lay a pine wreath on my brother's and father's graves. As I stood there in the cold, I was comforted by the feel of my dead sister's ring on my finger. When I returned to my mother's room, phone calls came from relatives in Switzerland to wish her well. My heart filled as she spoke the old Swiss–German dialect. But she quickly tired, and handed the phone to me. I fumbled for words; the language of my youth returned all too slowly. The transatlantic conversations connected the family but also reminded me of losses—my father, grandmothers, sister, and the severed family ties so common in immigrant families. I talked for nearly half an hour, first to one cousin, then to another. When I hung up, Mom complimented me on how well I did. I sensed she was giving me the responsibility of keeping our family together. I cried. In that brief moment, that half hour, that one day, all my past, present, and future losses converged.

Like Dorothy Becvar, I learned the hard way that life could be enriched by wrestling with loss and grief and the fact of one's own mortality. My own research has been about ambiguous losses, situations when someone we love is physically or psychologically missing, partly here yet partly gone, not clearly dead or alive. But I learned from real-life experiences that even in certified death, absolutes are rare. We hold on to ambiguity as hope that all is not lost when the heart stops.

From Elisabeth Kübler-Ross to James Agee, I have read about death in the family. But I learned about the folly of trying to "get over it" from experience—my 13-year-old brother's sudden death from bulbar polio the summer before the Salk vaccine came out; my sister's sudden death from lung cancer even though she did not smoke; my father's gradual death from advanced old age. Living in the presence of grief, to use Becvar's optimistic phrase, I learned that "getting over it" is not possible or desirable. I found I could hold the opposing ideas of absence and presence in my mind at the same time. I see this also in many of the couples and families with whom I work in therapy or research. Although some deaths are more ambiguous than others, all hold the possibility of some degree of presence in the lives of those left behind. You don't have to "get over it."

A subject as fearsome as death needs more than a didactic presentation. It begs for the experiential, which Dorothy Becvar gives us. She shares her own story about the sudden and needless death of her son and her subsequent journey toward acceptance, but not "closure," a word we both dislike. She lives concurrently with sorrow and joy. Dr. Becvar is an expert family systems theorist, but what pulled me into this book was her authority as a person who has "walked the walk." Her authority as a scholar is enriched by the authenticity of living in the presence of her own grief.

To blend personal and scholarly information about death, Dr. Becvar uses the narrative approach. But she does not simply tell us about narrative therapy, she shows us. Her stories and reflections touch both mind and heart to enrich our clinical skills and personal understanding.

Dr. Becvar's greatest gift, however, may be the information she gives us about the prevention of somatization in survivors even when the most difficult death occurs. From ancient Seneca to the latest research, she synthesizes a mountain of literature concerning the pragmatics, legalities, and emotional work before and after death occurs. She gives us an encyclopedic list of different types of death: children, adolescents, young adults, older adults, only children, men, women, pets, friends, fictive kin, same-sex partners, colleagues at work, fellow students, siblings, spouses, mothers, and fathers. While recommending a contextual approach for all, she makes the point repeatedly that each death, and each survivor's grief process, is unique. She gives us pragmatic information to help people reclaim joy after deaths that are anticipated, unexpected, euthanized, old, young, inside the family, or out. She gives us useful questions to help us face death. Throughout there is optimism; we can live with death: We can live—even have joy—in the presence of grief. Dorothy Becvar gives us just what we need to begin a much needed discourse.

In a culture that values youth and technology, talk about death is often shunned because it implies failure to heal, cure, fix, or solve; failure to win. As I have written, people who have the greatest need to control and master may have the most difficult time tolerating the ambiguity so inherent in loss and death. In a culture in which mastering problems is so highly prized, even assumed, we have much to learn about what lies ahead for all of us.

PAULINE BOSS, PhD
Professor and Family Therapist/Supervisor
University of Minnesota, St. Paul

Preface

When my 22-year-old son was killed in a bicycling accident in 1987, my world literally was shattered. I had lost one of my two precious children, a person I valued more than life itself. A remarkable young man—talented, vital, in perfect health, just entering the prime of life—was suddenly gone. My family was devastated and I was thrust into the realm of bereavement with no warning and very little prior experience. Until that time my only firsthand knowledge of death had come earlier in my life, through the loss of one classmate and three of my grandparents before I completed high school, and my remaining grandfather shortly after I graduated from college. Such was my acquaintance with grief. I also had been through a painful divorce and certainly had mourned the end of my first marriage 9 years previously. However, since then I had become happily remarried and had embarked on a whole new life, both personally and professionally. Although I had known moments of great sadness, for the most part mine had been basically a happy existence. I knew little about the agony of losing someone to whom I was deeply attached, and nothing in my life had prepared me adequately for the journey I was about to begin.

Unfortunately, as I have since learned, in our society a story such as mine is not uncommon. We fear death, we deny death, and all too often we do anything we can to avoid getting too close to it until we are confronted with the loss of a loved one. Therefore, we find ourselves somewhat uncertain as we attempt to respond to the pain others may be suffering and we are utterly bereft when the pain is our own. In the latter instance, the words of well-intentioned friends often add to our confusion and we find little public understanding of, or support for, the realities of our experience.

Over time, we recognize that the primary reality is that grief never really ends. Rather, each of us who has entered the "valley of the shadow of death" lives forever after, to one degree or another, in the presence of grief. More than picking up the pieces and moving on, we are challenged to create an entirely new picture, or story, about ourselves, about our world, about what it means to live. This challenge involves both acknowledging grief as a constant companion and at the same time learning once again to open ourselves up fully so that we may reclaim joy, as well as sadness, as a valid and acceptable part of our reality.

Given the enormity of such a challenge, it is easy to understand that meeting it may require a long period of time, and certainly far more than generally is deemed necessary or appropriate. However, the process of healing cannot be hurried. It also may require a great deal of energy and attention. Nor is there any one right way that healing *should* be pursued or completed. There is no magic formula and each person must be permitted to engage in the struggle to come to terms with death-related events and issues in a manner that is unique to and suitable for him or her.

Moreover, reaching a point of successful resolution does not necessarily mean "getting over" the loss. Indeed, for those who choose to play supportive roles in the lives of family members dealing with death, dying, bereavement, and related end-of-life issues, awareness of being in the presence of grief, regardless of how much time has passed, is crucial. Whether as a relative, friend, or professional, understanding that grief is an inevitable and ever-present part of the context may enhance the ability to provide meaningful assistance to others. Assuming grief, at least at some level, as a given, we then may move more productively to the search for whatever solutions are desired by those whom we wish to help.

Playing a supportive role also requires both an understanding of the realm of death, dying, and bereavement in a general sense and an awareness of the many ways in which death may enter the lives of those with whom we live and work. For a broader understanding in this regard, Part I of this book provides an overview of the varieties of the grief experience, or the contexts of grief. Considered, for example, is the fact that losing a parent is not the same as losing a child or a sibling. Similarly, we may learn that an anticipated death is different from one that occurs "out of the blue." Death from illness and death by suicide also provide sharply contrasting experiences for those who survive. And the process of dying, painful enough in and of itself, may be complicated immensely by the introduction of euthanasia considerations and issues.

At the same time, we cannot assume that the experience of a particular sort of death (e.g., of a parent) is the same for all people. Different kinds of relationships, differing backgrounds, divergent circumstances inevitably shape and color the meaning of each loss and may have long-term effects and ramifications that vary endlessly. Therefore, the first part of this book also presents many of the key issues about which to be mindful relative to each type of death. Always we are reminded of the importance of being sensitive to the unique needs, concerns, and level of involvement of each individual and each family.

Part I of this book draws many illustrations from the stories and experiences of clients, and each chapter concludes with a section on therapeutic conversations and reflections. The primary goal, however, is to provide a greater understanding of what may be going on for those who survive different kinds of loss. By contrast, in Part II we look more specifically at the therapeutic process and various issues of importance that may arise and need attention in this context. Thus, although the last three chapters also conclude with a section on therapeutic conversations and reflections, each chapter also offers specific strategies for helping clients who are bereaved. The focus in this section is thus grief in the context of therapy, or the common tasks with which clients are likely to be faced on the road to healing regardless of the type of loss suffered.

My own journey to healing has taken me along paths I barely knew existed, let alone previously had considered walking. In the process I often have strayed far from the traditional routes described by my former, now-discarded belief systems. Sometimes I have shocked not only my family members and friends but also myself. The going has not always been easy and unforeseen reactions continue to catch me by surprise. Nor do I believe that this journey has an ending. Although it has been more than 14 years, I know that I will never stop missing my son, or my parents, who in the last 12 years also have died.

I have been a fortunate traveler, however, and much support has been readily available to me along the way. I have an incredible network of family and friends who have "been there" since the beginning and who continue to provide comfort just by their presence. What is more, my work as a teacher and a family therapist has provided me with opportunities both to add professional wisdom to my personal experience and to be invited into the lives and stories of clients who also have been challenged by death, dying, bereavement, and related end-of-life issues. Many of these stories, as well as the understanding I have gained from them, will be shared with readers in the pages that follow.

Indeed, I have learned a great deal on my journey and there is much information and firsthand knowledge I wish to pass on to others. I understand, for example, how life may be enriched through the process of acknowledging and living in the awareness of our own mortality. I recognize how important it is to have a belief system that enables me to make sense of loss and grief despite the pain. Above all, I have lost my fear of death and I now consider it a great gift to be able to interact and work with others around issues related to the end of life. My greatest desire is that through this book I may provide a measure of hope and guidance for those who, like me, may be living and/or working in the presence of grief.

Acknowledgments

While writing a book is for me a labor of love, its completion would be far more difficult without the support of numerous others. I am extremely grateful to my editor, Kitty Moore, for her initial interest in the topic of death and dying; for her ability throughout the writing process to be available and interested without ever intruding; and for her affirmation and validation when the final product ultimately was delivered to her. I also wish to give thanks to the entire production staff of The Guilford Press, including copyeditor Lori Jacobs, Senior Production Editor Anna Brackett, and all the others unknown to me who share responsibility for having transformed my manuscript into this book.

I wish to acknowledge as well the debt of gratitude I feel toward the many students, clients, and colleagues with whom I have had the opportunity to work throughout my years as a teacher and a therapist. I have been both encouraged and enriched by our interactions and work together. As you have looked to me respectively with your passion for learning, your desire for healing, and your willingness to collaborate, I have been challenged to find ways to respond that might be most meaningful for each of you.

Finally, I could not have reached a place in my own life where writing this book was possible had it not been for the support of some other very special people in my world. To my wonderful friends—my "chosen" family—while you are too numerous to name, you know who you are and I want to say, once again, how fortunate I feel to be sharing my journey with you. To my brother Carl, I give thanks for understanding and being there all along the way. To my daughter, Lynne, your love and laughter and light are a continual source of unimaginable joy. To my husband, Ray, I feel truly blessed to have your absolute and unconditional love and support.

Contents

∾

xvii

Winter is come and gone,
But grief returns with the revolving year.

—PERCY BYSSHE SHELLEY

PART I

The Contexts of Grief

☙

CHAPTER 1

Introduction

❧

I struggled up the slope of Mount Evmandu to meet the famous guru of Nepsim, an ancient sage whose name I was forbidden to place in print. I was much younger then, but the long and arduous hike exhausted me, and, despite the cold, I was perspiring heavily when I reached the plateau where he made his home. He viewed me with a patient, almost amused, look, and I smiled wanly at him between attempts to gulp the thin air into my lungs. I made my way across the remaining hundred meters and slowly sat down on the ground—propping myself up against a large rock just outside his abode.

We were both silent for several minutes, and I felt the tension in me rise, then subside until I was calm. Perspiration prickled my skin, but the slight breeze was pleasantly cool, and soon I was relaxed. Finally I turned my head to look directly into the clear brown eyes, which were bright within his lined face. I realized that I would need to speak.

"Father," I said, "I need to understand something about what it means to die, before I can continue my studies." He continued to gaze at me with his open, bemused expression. "Father," I went on, "I want to know what a dying person feels when no one will speak with him, nor be open enough to permit him to speak, about his dying."

He was silent for three, perhaps four, minutes. I felt at peace because I knew he would answer. Finally, as though in the middle of a sentence, he said, "It is the horse on the dining-room table." We continued to gaze at each other for several minutes. I began to feel sleepy after my long journey, and I must have dozed off. When I woke up, he was gone, and the only activity was my own breathing.

I retraced my steps down the mountain—still feeling calm, knowing that his answer made me feel good, but not knowing why. I returned to my studies and gave no further thought to the event, not wishing to dwell upon it, yet secure that someday I should understand.

Many years later I was invited to the home of a casual friend for dinner. It was a modest house in a typical California development. The eight or ten other guests, people I did not know well, and I sat in the living room—drinking Safeway Scotch and bourbon and dipping celery sticks and raw cauliflower into a watery cheese dip. The conversation, initially halting, became more animated as we got to know each other and developed points of contact. The drinks undoubtedly also affected us.

Eventually the hostess appeared and invited us into the dining room for a buffet dinner. As I entered the room, I noticed with astonishment that a brown horse was sitting quietly on the dining-room table. Although it was small for a horse, it filled much of the large table. I caught my breath, but didn't say anything. I was the first one to enter, so I was able to turn, to watch the other guests. They responded much as I did—they entered and saw the horse, gasped or stared, but said nothing.

The host was the last to enter. He let out a silent shriek—looking rapidly from the horse to each of his guests with a wild stare. His mouth formed soundless words. Then in a voice choked with confusion he invited us to fill our plates from the buffet. His wife, equally disconcerted by what was clearly an unexpected horse, pointed to the name cards, which indicated where each of us was to sit.

The hostess led me to the buffet and handed me a plate. Others lined up behind me—each of us quiet. I filled my plate with rice and chicken and sat in my place. The others followed suit.

It was cramped, sitting there, trying to avoid getting too close to the horse, while pretending that no horse was there. My dish overlapped the edge of the table. Others found other ways to avoid physical contact with the horse. The host and hostess seemed as ill-at-ease as the rest of us. The conversation lagged. Every once in a while, someone would say something in an attempt to revive the earlier pleasant and innocuous discussion, but the overwhelming presence of the horse so filled our thoughts that talk of taxes or politics or the lack of rain seemed inconsequential.

Dinner ended, and the hostess brought coffee. I can recall everything on my plate and yet have no memory of having eaten. We drank in silence—all of us trying not to look at the horse, yet unable to keep our eyes or thoughts anywhere else.

I thought several times of saying, "Hey, there's a horse on the dining-room table." But I hardly knew the host, and I didn't wish to embarrass him by mentioning something that obviously discomforted him at least as much as it disconcerted me. After all, it was his house. And what do you say to a man with a horse on his dining-room table? I could have said that I did not mind, but that was not true—its presence upset me so much that I enjoyed neither the dinner nor the company. I could have said that I knew how difficult it was to have a horse on one's dining-room table, but that wasn't true either; I had no idea. I could have said something like, "How do you feel about having a horse on your dining-room table?", but I didn't want to sound like a psychologist. Perhaps, I thought, if I ignore it, it will go away. Of course I knew that it wouldn't. It didn't.

I later learned that the host and hostess were hoping the dinner would be a success in spite of the horse. They felt that to mention it would make us so uncomfortable that we wouldn't enjoy our visit—of course we didn't enjoy the evening anyway. They were fearful that we would try to offer them sympathy, which they didn't want, or understanding, which they needed but could not accept. They wanted the party to be a success, so they decided to try to make the evening as enjoyable as possible. But it was apparent that they—like their guests—could think of little else than the horse.

I excused myself shortly after dinner and went home. The evening had been terrible. I never wanted to see the host and hostess again, although I was eager to seek out the other guests and learn what they felt about the occasion. I felt confused about what had happened and extremely tense. The evening had been grotesque. I was careful to avoid the host and hostess after that, and I did my best to stay away altogether from the neighborhood.

Recently I visited Nepsim again. I decided to seek out the guru once more. He was still alive, although nearing death, and he would speak only to a few. I repeated my journey and eventually found myself sitting across from him.

Once again I asked, "Father, I want to know what a dying person feels when no one will speak with him, nor be open enough to permit him to speak, about his dying."

The old man was quiet, and we sat without speaking for nearly an hour. Since he did not bid me leave, I remained. Although I was content, I feared he would not share his wisdom, but he finally spoke. The words came slowly.

"My son, it is the horse on the dining-room table. It is a horse that visits every house and sits on every dining-room table—the tables of the rich and of the poor, of the simple and of the wise. This horse just sits there, but its presence makes you wish to leave without speaking of it. If you leave, you will always fear the presence of the horse. When it sits on your table, you will wish to speak of it, but you may not be able to.

"However, if you speak about the horse, then you will find that others can also speak about the horse—most others, at least, if you are gentle and kind as you speak. The horse will remain on the dining-room table, but you will not be so distraught. You will enjoy your repast, and you will enjoy the company of the *host and hostess. Or, if it is your table, you will enjoy the presence of your guests. You cannot make magic to have the horse disappear, but you can speak of the horse and thereby render it less powerful."*

The old man then rose and, motioning me to follow, walked slowly to his hut. "Now we shall eat," he said quietly. I entered the hut and had difficulty adjusting to the dark. The guru walked to a cupboard in the corner and took out some bread and some cheese, which he placed on a mat. He motioned to me to sit and share his food. I saw a small horse sitting quietly in the center of the mat. He noticed this and said, "That horse need not disturb us." I thoroughly enjoyed the meal. Our discussion lasted far into the night, while the horse sat there quietly throughout our time together.

—RICHARD KALISH (1985)

UNDERSTANDING DEATH, DYING, AND BEREAVEMENT

To understand fully what it means to be in the presence of grief we must speak of death. And to speak of death is to enter the realm of the supreme mystery, that of the unanswerable question. For although it certainly is the most inevitable fact of life, death also represents the quintessential paradox: "From the very beginning we sense the oxymoronic quality of death. Death is destroyer and redeemer; the ultimate cruelty and the essence of release; universally feared but sometimes actively sought; undeniably ubiquitous, yet incomprehensibly unique; of all phenomena, the most obvious and the least reportable, feared yet fascinating" (Shneidman, 1980a, p. 10).

Death may indeed be fascinating. However, more commonly it is feared. Thus, as we begin the pursuit of greater awareness for ourselves and an enhanced ability to work with others in the realm of death, dying, bereavement, and related end-of-life issues, the first task generally involves becoming acquainted and comfortable with "the horse on the dining-room table," the fact that each of us ultimately must die. The degree to which this may or may not be a challenge will be influenced significantly both by the stories and experiences each of us brings with us from our families of origin and by the rules and norms, or "culture tales" (Howard, 1991), of the society in which we live.

We all received from our families a variety of messages, both implicit and explicit, about whether death was to be considered an uninvited stranger or a welcome guest. There is a good chance, however, that previously we may not have focused on bringing these messages into conscious awareness. Therefore, it is a good idea to take a few moments to consider our first encounter with death and dying. Was it through the loss of a grandparent, parent, sibling, other family member, friend, stranger, public figure, pet? What was the reaction and how did those around us respond? Other questions we may wish to ask ourselves include the following: How was the subject of death in general talked about or handled by the people with whom we grew up? What was the story about death and what happens after we die that we told ourselves as children and how has this story evolved and changed over the years? What events and people have been involved in the creation of our story about death and dying? How have we been influenced by our reading, the media, religious beliefs, our own health, the death of someone close? Have you thought about your own death or when and how you might die or might prefer to die? What are the feelings we experience when we consider and confront our own mortality?

Responding to these questions may enable us to get in touch more fully with our personal beliefs about death and dying as well as with the process of their creation. As we respond, we must be aware that our answers may be revealing and may have consequences that go far beyond the desire to gain intellectual knowledge. Although many would consider a focus on concerns such as these to be rather morbid, others would urge us to recognize the extent to which life may be enhanced by a full consideration of death-related issues (Sogyal, 1992).

In this regard it may be important as well to remember that for any concept to have meaning, a second concept which is a logical complement to the first also is required. Thus, for example, we are able to understand the concept of happy as we distinguish it from the concept of sad. Similarly, sweet would be difficult to comprehend without being able to contrast it with sour. This is the challenge experienced by those born without sight as they struggle to make sense of colors without the visual ability to compare, for example, red and blue. As Bateson (1972) noted many years ago, it is through the relationships of difference that meaningful information is communicated. And so it is with life and death; each requires the other and without both, neither would be a meaningful concept.

However, as we exist in a particular social context, we tend to imbue the sides of each set of complementarities, or opposite concepts, with negative and positive connotations. Despite the fact that happy is not necessarily better than sad, nor sweet better than sour, any more than blue is better than red, we make value judgments consistent with our preferences and forget that it is we who have created the story that sad and sour are negative experiences. Although this is by no means a universal response, certainly in our culture the attribution of negativity is the typical reaction to death.

Indeed, despite some shifts in recent years in our attitude toward death and dying, we live in a society in which denial (Becker, 1973) and fear (Foos-Graber, 1989) continue to be the norm. We attempt to push thoughts of death out of our awareness at every opportunity and when we are unsuccessful we often find ourselves feeling frightened and lost. So negative is our perception that death often is construed as a social disease (Shneidman, 1980a), thus making it a less acceptable topic of conversation than is sexual activity (Gorer, 1980). And even when we allow ourselves to engage in discourse about death, we tend to do so in a solemn and subdued manner (Hainer, 1997, p. 1D), thereby enhancing its fearfulness and heightening our anxiety.

Perhaps it would be appropriate to become aware of and to consider critically the statement, however unintended, we may be making as our stance toward death is basically one of trepidation. As Plato writes in his *Apology*: "For the fear of death is indeed the pretense of wisdom, and not real wisdom, being a pretense of knowing the unknown; and no one knows whether death, which men in their fear apprehend to be the greatest evil, may not be the greatest good" (in Packard, 1981, p. 9).

In fact, we do not know that death is something evil. Nevertheless, as we engage in a search today for definitions we find that, according to the dictionary, death refers not only to the loss or destroyer of life, and to extinction, but also to anything so dreadful as to seem like death. Further, death often is symbolized by a skeleton with a scythe, the grim reaper. We therefore may find it difficult even to say the word and thus we hear that someone has "passed," or gone to his or her "great reward." More colloquially some common terms to describe the fact that someone has died include "kicked the bucket" or "bought the farm."

The reality is that most of our public associations with death appear to be anything but positive. It therefore follows that we are fearful and not only avoid the topic but also engage, sometimes fanatically, in activities aimed at prolonging life and denying death. For example, we value a youthful rather than a mature appearance. Unless or until pressed by necessity we put off discussions about the kind of funeral we might like, where and how we would prefer to die, and what our wishes are in terms of burial. We delay the making of a will, or thinking about a living will.

And once death has arrived, we support the practice of embalming in an attempt to create a life-like appearance for the one who has died. According to Aries (1980), however, embalming is virtually unheard of in Europe. Further, it is his belief that in the United States it is the ultimate attempt to maintain the facade of life, and thereby to deny the reality of death.

Consistent with such an attitude, both as individuals and as a society, we also devote enormous amounts of time, money, and energy to efforts aimed at sustaining life. We permit the use of extreme measures of life support for the dying, even after all hope of recovery has ceased. And we often refuse to let our loved ones go, emotionally, even when their time seems to have come. However, the main emphasis of these efforts generally tends to be on quantity rather than on quality. The irony here is that the goal of a rich and full life, despite its length, may perhaps best be achieved in the context of full awareness and acceptance of death. As Norman Cousins (1989) writes,

> Hope, faith, love, and a strong will to live offer no promise of immortality, only proof of our uniqueness as human beings and the opportunity to experience full growth even under the grimmest circumstances. The clock provides only a technical measurement of how long we live. Far more real than the ticking of time is the way we open up the minutes and invest them with meaning. Death is not the ultimate tragedy in life. The ultimate tragedy is to die without discovering the possibilities of full growth. The approach of death need not be denial of that growth. (p. 25)

As we seek to avert the tragedy of which Cousins speaks and to engage in the process of living more fully, or of "befriending our death" (Nouwen, 1994), we may actually enhance our relationships with ourselves, with those around us, and with our world. As we live in the awareness that we begin to die as soon as we are born, each moment becomes a gift to be cherished. Life, with all its opportunities for growth and learning, becomes a treasure to be handled with care. And the people with whom we share our lives become special in entirely new ways. We recognize the importance of not squandering our riches, of spending our time wisely. Along the way, we also may become better equipped to be with and help others as we model for them what is possible through acknowledgment that we are indeed finite creatures.

This process of acknowledgment, of *learning to accept and to live with*, is the essence of what is meant by the term "resolve," the understanding of which is the goal of this book: helping family members to successfully *resolve* death, dying, bereavement, and related end-of-life issues. However, that which we must resolve, or learn to accept and live with, changes as death moves from being an abstract concept to a concrete reality. To explain, as we seek on the one hand to come to terms with our own mortality, our greatest challenges may emerge from feelings such as fear of the unknown, concerns about those whom we would be leaving, disappointment about what we have not accomplished, or despair that this may be all there is. On the other hand, the death of a loved one catapults us into an entirely different realm, one characterized by equally significant but different kinds of issues and challenges.

Indeed, one of the foremost realities, and perhaps the greatest paradox, that often emerges when we lose someone we love is the fact that we also may lose our fear of death. We even may lose our will to live. In this instance, therefore, resolving, or coming to terms with death, may involve not only learning to accept and live with pain but also finding ways to answer some of life's biggest questions: "Who am I?" "Why am I here?" "What is life all about?" "Is it worth the effort?" We may be challenged to create meaning where none seems to exist. We may find ourselves at sea without the anchor of previously cherished and long-held beliefs. All the basic tenets which have been the ground of our being, the foundation on which we have built our lives, may have been washed away as we discovered that they were insufficient to sustain us in our time of greatest need. And even when this is not the case, we often are faced with the task of figuring out how to continue to live in a much altered context.

Clearly, however, not all encounters with death and dying will have consequences with the magnitude of those just described. Some of the most crucial factors influencing the impact of the loss, as well as the ability of those who survive to cope, include the dimension of time, the family position and life stages of the people involved, the intensity or closeness of relationships, and the manner in which both dying and death have occurred. Thus, even within one family the experience of a death will be unique for each different family member. Those who desire to assist family members, therefore, must be sensitive to the particular configuration of circumstances that characterize the context of each individual's grief experience.

The dimension of time is significant in many ways and has important ramifications for both the dying and for those who survive. As will become apparent, neither unanticipated nor anticipated death is necessarily more to be desired and both kinds of experience have their share of benefits and losses. Similarly, the age of the person at the time of death is worthy of attention but no one age inevitably means that the survivors will have an easier time handling the loss. Rather, the effect of time must be considered relative to the variety of other factors which also may influence the grieving process for each person involved and affected. In the following sections we introduce some of the particular ways in which the dimension of time may have an impact.

WHEN DEATH COMES UNANNOUNCED

When death is unanticipated, or comes without warning, there is no time for anyone to prepare for what has happened. In this case, the person who has died may have made no arrangements or may have had no opportunity to express his or her wishes regarding issues such as organ donation, funeral arrangements, and burial preferences. There may be many loose ends around financial and legal issues. What may be even more critical, however, is the sense of dislocation and incongruity experienced by the survivors. One moment the person was alive and healthy; the next moment the person is gone forever. Also important in this regard is the lack of closure the survivor may be experiencing. There has been no time for farewells and guilt may emerge regarding unresolved conflicts or dissatisfaction about things left undone or unsaid.

Accordingly, acute feelings of unreality, disbelief, and shock are common in the aftermath of a sudden and unexpected death. Dissonance in terms of basic assumptions and meaning systems is highly likely, particularly if the death occurred under tragic circumstances or involved the loss of a child. In the latter instance, the feeling of a death out of time is extremely significant (Gilbert, 1997). In the event of a violent or wrongful death, anger and frustration at the injustice may be added to grief over the loss.

At the same time, when death comes unannounced, and particularly if it is instantaneous, there may be some sense of gratitude that the person did not suffer, or died doing something she or he loved, or in the midst of a full and active life. Thus, for example, the parents of soldiers killed in battle often have found solace in the thought that their child gave up her or his life in the service of a country all hold dear. Although this may be of small comfort in the moment, it may ease the pain of the loss as time enables the survivors to view the event from a less anguished perspective. In retrospect there even may be relief that the person who died did not have to experience subsequent hardships which may have been inevitable

had she or he lived. All these factors contrast sharply with events surrounding a death that is more or less expected.

WHEN DEATH IS ANTICIPATED

In the case of an anticipated death, the dying person often is provided
with an opportunity to put his or her affairs in order, to tie up loose ends,
so to speak. There is time to create a will, if necessary or desired, and to
indicate personal preferences about issues such as dying at home or in a
hospital as well as about measures that are or are not to be taken to sustain
life. There is time to consider the possibility of organ donation and to participate in funeral arrangements and burial decisions. There is time as
well to achieve closure in significant relationships, a process which may
be facilitated by the imminence of death. There also is an opportunity for
everyone involved to assimilate what is happening, to realign beliefs if appropriate or necessary, and to make plans for a future without the person
who is dying.

At the same time, having foreknowledge also tends to initiate a period of anticipatory mourning in which everyone involved is faced with
the inevitability of the loss. In this case, the grieving process may begin
even though the death has not yet occurred (Rolland, 1991). In the event
of an extended dying process, significant stress also may be placed on
caretakers, who may feel angry and/or overwhelmed by the situation. In
addition, a sense of remorse about being a burden may emerge on the part
of the person who is dying. Attempts to resolve conflicts also may prove
futile, leading to feelings of frustration for those involved. When the
death ultimately occurs, survivors may experience a complex set of emotions including sadness about the loss, gratitude that suffering has ended
for the dying person, relief that there will now be a respite for the caregivers, and guilt about what are perfectly normal, if mixed, reactions.
What is more, the desire to alleviate emotional and physical pain during a
period of extended dying may have opened the door to another set of end-
of-life issues with long-lasting ramifications.

WHEN THE QUESTION OF EUTHANASIA EMERGES

An additional factor that may emerge in the context of anticipated death
involves questions about the rights of people to consider and choose the

manner and timing of their own death. Since the late 1990s, much heated controversy has been captured by the media as we have debated publicly such questions as when it is appropriate for life-support systems to be removed, how much suffering, both physical and emotional, a person should have to endure, the ramifications of the use of narcotics which may relieve physical pain but dull consciousness, and the appropriateness of allowing a person to die by refusing food and liquids (Peay, 1997). As we attempt to assist family members who may be seeking, in a very personal manner, answers to questions such as these, we must be cognizant of both legal and professional responsibilities (Becvar, 2000a). We also must be sensitive to the ways in which families may be torn apart as they endeavor to cope with this dimension of the dying process. Indeed, many controversies may surface regarding whose right it is to make what decision and how differences of opinion are to be handled in the midst of efforts to cope with the fact that a loved one not only is dying but that it promises to be a long, slow, and painful process. And all these debates are further influenced by the roles and ages of those involved at the time of death.

WHEN A CHILD DIES

Whether death has been unanticipated or has occurred in some configuration of the circumstances associated with anticipated death, the family position and life stages of the people participating, and particularly of the person who is dying or has died, also have a tremendous influence on the way in which the event is experienced. Nowhere is this more evident than when a child dies. Regardless of other variables, the death of one's own child almost always seems a travesty. There is an extreme sense of dissonance and a feeling of something being extraordinarily wrong when parents bury a son or daughter. This is especially true in the current era in which a continually increasing life expectancy seems to promise a full and active existence well into our 70s and 80s. Thus, the death of a child may seem even more unlikely than in an earlier era when disease regularly claimed the lives of many at a young age. And even if the child is not our own, there appears to be something inordinately wrong or unfair about having life cut short. What is more, regardless of the fact that the person who died was an adult, the loss for parents generally continues to be excruciating as they simply don't expect to outlive their children. Indeed, there is probably no way that one can be prepared adequately for or can be expected to accept easily the death of a child.

WHEN A SIBLING DIES

Similarly, siblings may be totally unprepared to handle the death of a brother or sister, even after a prolonged illness. With no past experience, young children may not have a way of understanding either what has happened or the impact of this event on their parents. If they are older, the intensity of their experience often is overlooked (Becvar, 2000b) even though they may be feeling an enormous amount of grief. Further, if they are adults, they even may be called on to take over for their parents (Nolen-Hoeksema & Larson, 1999). Thus, they may be asked to handle the details of funeral arrangements or the logistics involved with housing and feeding relatives from out of town. However, the death of a sibling represents the severing of an extremely important connection. It may mean the loss of a beloved companion, mentor, or protector. It also makes real the awareness of one's own vulnerability and mortality. As a function of such a loss, siblings may be moved to change their attitudes about career choices, family relationships, and the importance of creating a healthy lifestyle. At the same time, they may find themselves feeling like an "endangered species" as their parents become extremely overprotective out of fear that they may lose another child, and/or they may feel bereft of parents, as the latter are now totally absorbed in their own grief. And while this is occurring, the child has fewer or no siblings to whom to turn for support in significantly changed circumstances.

WHEN A PARENT DIES

A more expected occurrence for siblings is the death of a parent. In the natural order of things we presume that we will outlive our mothers and fathers. Nevertheless, when a parent dies, it signifies the end of a primary attachment bond and therefore the loss of one of the most important relationships in our lives. No matter what the age at which one loses a parent, and while different developmental issues thus may emerge (Shapiro, 1994), life thereafter is forever altered. What is more, the degree of closeness or distance characterizing the relationship with the deceased parent apparently has little influence on the intensity of the grief experienced by surviving children (Umberson & Chen, 1994). More crucial, perhaps, is the time of life at which death occurs. That is, we certainly don't anticipate that our parents will die before they have reached a ripe old age or while we are still young. Indeed, the younger the child, the greater may be the long-term consequences of the death of a parent. The reality is that with each milestone passed following the death of a parent, her or his absence once again is brought into sharper focus. Not being able to share graduations, weddings, the birth of a baby, and other significant events with the parent who has died lends a bittersweet taste to otherwise happy occasions. Thus, once again we also must be sensitive to the dimensions of role and life stage and to issues related to the disruption occasioned by a death "out of time."

WHEN A SPOUSE DIES

When a spouse or partner in a committed relationship dies, similar issues emerge as a function of the age at the time of death, thereby changing the complexion of the loss. For example, the experience of widowhood varies considerably for young adults and/or those with young children, as compared with those in midlife or old age. The expectation is that the members of the couple will grow old together and thus a death in youth or in the middle of life is likely to be more of a shock. In all situations, however, when a wife, husband, or partner dies one loses one's companion and counterpart and the feelings of aloneness may be overwhelming. Even in the case of a relationship characterized by conflict, the absence of someone with whom to discuss and perhaps commiserate about daily events, the loss of a sexual partner, the lack of someone to share responsibilities for home and family, the burdens associated with being a single parent, as well as concerns about financial security, all may be keenly felt. And the sense of aloneness may be exacerbated as couple friends drift away, failing to include the now single person in formerly shared activities. Over time, as the widow or widower begins to consider establishing a new committed relationship, she or he also may be assailed by feelings of guilt or betrayal of the spouse or partner who has died. What is more, depending on gender, age, and the presence or absence of children, opportunities to create such a new relationship may be limited. The idea of starting over with another person, let alone confusion about how to proceed, also may seem overwhelming. Although spouses or partners are not related by blood, the closeness and intertwining of lives which characterize the marital or committed relationship may make the death of a spouse or partner an extraordinary challenge.

WHEN AN EXTENDED FAMILY MEMBER
OR FRIEND DIES

Different kinds of challenges may arise with the death of an extended family member or friend. In this case the grief experienced may go unacknowledged as attention is focused primarily on immediate family members. For example, there certainly is little provision for absence from work in such situations. Therefore, although a person may be grieving, she or he may fail to give adequate consideration to her or his own needs and may not take time to facilitate the process of healing. What is more, the effort to provide support for those who seemingly are most closely affected also may be difficult as this person attempts both to be of assistance and to avoid intruding. Indeed, the fact that one is not part of the inner circle may make it hard to know what would be considered helpful. And despite one's sadness, there also may be relief or gratitude that it was not one's own family member, or even oneself, who has been struck down.

At the same time, the kinds of reactions just described often are followed by a sense of guilt for having had the feelings. Or, conversely, one may wonder why the particular person was the one to die rather than oneself or one's own family member. And certainly issues regarding one's own mortality may rise to the surface through the contemplation of death from a somewhat removed perspective.

Clearly, with the death of an extended family member or friend, as with the deaths of people in each of the various roles and life stages previously mentioned, an extremely important variable is the intensity or closeness of relationships. We cannot assume more or less grief based on the degree of kinship. For example, one may have had a much deeper and more meaningful relationship with a devoted uncle than one had with a parent. Similarly, in this era of extreme mobility and loosening of family ties, the loss of a friend may have much greater significance than does the death of someone to whom we are related by blood.

As we also have touched on briefly, the manner in which both the dying and the death have occurred plays an important part in the bereavement process. Death following an extended illness, sudden or accidental death, violent or wrongful death, death by suicide, and ambiguous death and loss lend different meanings and have different impacts on the grief experience. The manner of death also may greatly influence how funerals and other ceremonies are handled. In the case of a suicide, for example, the family may wish to keep the funeral small and private. What is more, there may be limited awareness of the variety of options available relative to the creation of funerals and other rituals, both formal and informal. Thus, one of the ways in which we may be of assistance is through the process of helping family members to understand the importance of honoring the person who has died in ways that are not only respectful of that person's wishes but also helpful and healing for those who survive.

CREATING FUNERALS, CEREMONIES, AND OTHER HEALING RITUALS

Given a general reluctance to broach the subject of death and dying, particularly our own, it is not surprising that most people have not delved too deeply into the business of funeral arrangements much before it becomes an absolute necessity. And even when preplanning is engaged in, typically we tend to assume that the process will be consistent with the norms of our society. Thus, we may choose either burial or cremation, we might designate our preference for type of service or ritual, we may select the music if there is to be any. We might even decide to become an organ donor or to donate our body to science. We also may purchase a cemetery lot and design and/or order a tombstone. But rarely do we stop to consider significant deviations from the norm. When death arrives, a fairly standard script typically is followed.

Accordingly, we as survivors tend to have little or nothing to do with the final preparation of the body and very little actual contact with the person once she or he has died. When next we see the deceased, often in the context of a viewing, visitation, or wake, she or he has been embalmed, dressed, and made up with cosmetics in an attempt to have him or her look as life-like as possible. Although we may have interacted with morticians and clergypersons in order to handle formal details, there is no sense of having experienced in a more informal, personal manner the transition of the loved one following death. And this lack of closure may add to our grief and confusion.

Next, we most likely find ourselves attending a funeral service—in a religious context, at the funeral home, or by the grave site. Although we may have indicated preferences and had a hand in the planning, once again the ritual usually is presided over by an "outsider"—the official representative of our particular religious or spiritual community. However, active participation on the part of the bereaved most often is constrained by tradition. What is more, the entire funeral process generally is completed in 1 to 3 days.

Although many certainly will continue to prefer to adhere to the common tradition, and in fact might be horrified by the thought of any deviation from it, others may find the opportunity to engage in a hands-on manner in the after-death preparations of the body as well as in the funeral and burial a balm for the wound of grief and an important catalyst for the healing process. Involvement in preparation of the body can range from being included in what is taking place at the mortuary to handling and preparing the body entirely on one's own. In terms of the funeral service, family members may choose to take on some of the primary roles in the prescribed ritual, or they may take total responsibility for the creation of a ceremony.

It is important for those who desire greater participation to be aware of actual legal limitations and regulations for the area in which the death has occurred or the funeral is to take place. Inasmuch as we as a society have turned over most of the responsibility for those who have died to the profession of funeral directors, we as individuals may be surprised to learn how much leeway actually exists. And whereas the violation of tradition may at first seem overwhelming, it is important to be sensitive to the degree to which the bereavement process may be facilitated as survivors are able to do something meaningful—to express their caring, feel a sense of control, and engage in a personally fulfilling farewell ceremony for the one who has died.

Regardless of the type of funeral or ceremony, however, part of the distress experienced by the bereaved in the days, weeks, and months that follow arises from the interruption of the repetitive patterns of interaction which have provided a sense of security in one's life and world. From the most mundane rituals, such as preparing meals or sharing conversations, to the family traditions surrounding major holidays and celebrations, one is faced with a lack of consistency and predictability. Inevitably, attention must be given to finding new routines, new ways to manage daily as well as seasonal or major milestone-marking events.

The task may seem difficult or even overwhelming at first, but revising old traditions may become an important part of the healing journey. Creating ways to acknowledge the one who has died may facilitate more open communication among family members. Rituals also may help with the task of managing a new event occasioned by the loss, that of the anniversary of the death. Indeed, even many years later, when one is not particularly conscious of the date, it can have an impact on how one feels or behaves. It therefore may be useful to plan to honor and acknowledge the day in a deliberate manner. Taking time off from work, making a trip to a favorite place, visiting the cemetery, or preparing and eating the food that was most enjoyed by the loved one are but a few ideas that may prove beneficial in this regard. As I have emphasized, life in the presence of grief is new and different and honoring that difference through ritual may make its painful aspects more bearable as one attempts to recreate a meaningful existence.

BEREAVEMENT AND THE SEARCH FOR MEANING

After the funeral or other ceremony, and particularly if there has not been a significant sense of completion, the survivors may find themselves plunged much more intensely into the experience of grief. In the immediate aftermath of the death they may have been caught up in the details of making various arrangements. They may have been flooded with phone calls, cards, visits, and the presence of relatives and close friends. Most likely, they have not had to deal with day-to-day cares and concerns (e.g., meal preparations or laundry). Although there may have been great pain, there often has been little time or energy for deep thought or soul-searching reflection.

Once the last guest goes home, however, the bereaved person is faced with the awareness that while life around him or her continues to go on in normal ways, normal no longer has much meaning. It is perhaps jarring to see people laughing and having a good time, seemingly without a care in the world. It feels ridiculous to be worried about paying bills or fixing a leaky faucet. If staying home from work is not an option, doing the job may become a process of going through the motions with little care about what is being done. The bereaved person may go to a store to purchase something but once inside wonder why she or he came. Feelings of numbness alternating with the constant need to cry may characterize this initial phase of mourning.

For many the ability to cope effectively and move beyond this phase may hinge on the degree to which they are able to make sense out of or find meaning in what has transpired; that is, we humans are a theory-building, meaning-making species. We need stories or explanations to help us understand the events in our world. Most often, we search for the answer to the question, "Why?" We tend to believe that problems can be solved through exploration into and insight about their cause. However, although knowledge of the cause of death may be available to us, the reason for the person's death often is not. And even when we can see that it makes sense, for example, that the heart of an elderly person simply has given out, that it was his or her time to die, we may be surprised to find ourselves unable to be consoled by ideas or concepts in which we thought we believed.

Further, if the death is an example of a bad thing happening to a good person (Kushner, 1981), we may find the search for meaning even more challenging. That is, we may have a much harder time coming up with explanations that provide solace in the midst of great grief for a "death out of time," for accidental or violent death, for suicide. And despite the best intentions on the part of well-meaning family members or friends, phrases such as "God doesn't give us any burden we can't bear," or "only the good die young" may not soothe the bereaved spirit. Indeed, this may be so even though the recipient of the message previously may have believed in or spoken such phrases to others. Further, concepts which are foreign or strange may add to the confusion rather than provide assistance. For example, the ideas that one day the person might "thank God for what has happened," or that "each of us chooses the time and manner of our death," although meaningful in the context of some belief systems, are merely noise in the context of others.

Finding or making meaning is a personal process, one that can be supported and facilitated but ultimately must be accomplished in the way that is most appropriate for each person. Those who seek to help may be most effective when they are able to provide time, space, and encouragement for exploration. Offering to be a sounding board or to share one's own journey also may be useful as long as there is no insistence on one right way or path to follow. Although it may seem like a daunting challenge, at least initially, the goal ultimately is to facilitate for the bereaved the creation of a reality that includes not only sadness but also joy.

RECLAIMING JOY

Just as a death inevitably marks the end of one of life's chapters, it also signifies the beginning of a new one. This new chapter may be unwelcome and strange but it also has the capacity to open doors to greater awareness, enhanced sensitivity, and increased compassion. It may even lead us to greater wisdom:

> Wisdom is often born in the shadows, frequently more visible in the darkness than the light. The stadium lights of knowledge that seek to eliminate

natural cycles of night and day, death and rebirth, sorrow and joy do not cast shadows—they provide only the steady glare of illumination. We must move into darker places if we are to find the wisdom we so desperately need. We rarely go there willingly, though every life contains its own cycles of grief and celebration. To meet wisdom in these dark places we must be willing and able to hold all of what life gives us, to exclude nothing of ourselves or the world, to tell ourselves the truth. Wisdom will stretch us far beyond where we thought we could or wanted to go. She will show us what we cannot change or control, reveal what is hard to know about ourselves and the world, and tear at the illusions of what we think we know, until we are surrounded by the vastness of the mystery. (Dreamer, 1999, p. 41)

Although those of us who choose to be with and support bereaved family members or clients may not be able to share this perception at the outset, we can keep it in mind and allow it to permeate and color our responses. We, too, can learn to live in two realities: As we encourage in others the ability to understand that the reality of grief does not preclude the possibility of also being happy, we can acknowledge explicitly the pain that others may be feeling while simultaneously having knowledge about the potential to reclaim joy that is also part of the experience. Ideally the creation of such a stance will be facilitated by exploring more deeply in the following chapters each of the topics touched on briefly in this introductory overview.

THERAPEUTIC CONVERSATIONS AND REFLECTIONS

∾

Many years ago my assistance was requested by a family in which the youngest of seven adult children, a young woman in her mid-20s, had been diagnosed with a terminal illness and was nearing death. We spent our first evening together gathered in the living room of the family home. Both parents as well as all their offspring were present. And all those who were married also had brought their spouses, so we were somewhat crowded, which I am sure was not at all unusual for such a large family.

After the introductions had been made, I asked someone to talk about why I had been invited and what the family wanted to ac-
(cont.)

---

complish. The oldest son answered, saying that he was expressing the hope, shared by all his siblings and their spouses, that the family members would be able to talk about what was happening, let their sister know how much she was loved and supported, and provide a forum to speak about death and dying now and in the future.

The young woman who was dying then spoke quite eloquently about how thankful she was to have such a loving, caring support system. She expressed her gratitude for the willingness of her family members to come together as they were and for all the help and support she already had been receiving. And she also spoke about her deeply religious convictions and about the fact that she felt at peace with the reality that she was dying. She was not angry at God or fate, nor was she looking for a miracle. She was ready to leave when the time came.

Many of the young woman's siblings expressed both frustration with and, at the same time, understanding for their sister. They wished she would fight harder, try more experimental drugs. But they also knew she was tired and they respected her refusal of further treatment. Indeed, what eventually emerged was the fact that the underlying motive that had precipitated the meeting really had much more to do with what they feared would happen after she died than it did with their acceptance of her death.

As recounted by one of the younger siblings, they had also had another sister. She had been the second oldest child and had died many years previously—killed in an automobile accident during her senior year in high school. The feelings shared by the siblings were that their parents had never recovered fully from this event and that the family had never been the same since that time.

Although the children acknowledged that their parents had done all the necessary things for them, they felt that something basic had been lost. Their perception was that their parents had left them emotionally. What is more, they had not been permitted to speak about the changes, to talk about their sister, or even to discuss death and dying in a general way. Most felt a great deal of anger about what had happened and they wanted to prevent further damage from occurring when their youngest sister died. It was clear that they valued the family relationships and they also wanted to use the present tragedy to facilitate the healing of some of the old wounds.

The willingness of everyone to participate spoke to me immediately about the strengths and capacity for rebuilding relationships within this family. What is more, rather than becoming defensive, the parents were able to acknowledge and finally speak about the devastation they had experienced when their older daughter died. They seemed to welcome the opportunity to be able to express verbally their sadness relative to both their daughters. And they apologized to all their children for their previous inability to meet all of their needs, particularly at an emotional level. They knew that they had been both distant and fearful and yet could not seem to change.

The children, in turn, appreciated their parents' response and recognized that they had done the best they could. Rather than spending a lot of time with blame and anger, they were more interested now in avoiding the repetition of past mistakes and in doing a better job of dealing with the death of their younger sister. And that is the direction in which therapy ultimately proceeded with very beneficial outcomes.

What struck me then, as it does now, is the potential for either greater devastation or great healing that may occur when a loved one dies. With every crisis comes both challenge and opportunity, and when the crisis is precipitated by a death, the capacity for destruction as well as creation is increased geometrically. If there is meaningful support, if there is permission to speak, if there is a context of sensitivity and understanding, everyone stands to gain in spite of the loss. When these elements are missing, the damage done may be severe.

However, as the family in this instance illustrates, even after many years much healing remains possible. Although the past certainly was not able to be erased, a restorying which allowed each person to give voice to her or his respective feelings, both then and now, changed significantly the meaning associated with previous events. It also enabled a sense of greater solidarity as parents and siblings together participated with and supported their daughter/sister throughout her dying in the present and began the process of learning to live without her in the future.

CHAPTER 2

Understanding Death, Dying, and Bereavement

∾

I have begun to think that life on earth is the least portion of "life." Believing as I do that my child is with God and that there is eternal life makes me think that perhaps we endow this piece of life, which is so brief relative to eternity, with more importance than it deserves. Or perhaps we tend to cling to it more desperately than is appropriate. Certainly I have done that in the past. But, for me, part of that was not wanting to miss out on my children's lives. And now all of that has changed.

—DSB

*   *   *

I have spent the day wondering which is life and which is death. It occurs to me that life as we know it might, from the perspective of another reality, be death. That is, could it be that we are born into this reality at the end of life in a previous reality?

—DSB

*   *   *

I have a very deep curiosity about <u>where</u> my husband really is. I know his body is at the cemetery. But my lifetime Christian beliefs are now put to the test. Where is he? Does he know my thoughts? Does he know how much we miss him? Did he see our children graduate? Does he know our son is having a rough time? Can he see the basement has been remodeled? Our other son's apartment? Our daughter's tears? The friends who keep us going? He loved the rain and storms; is <u>all</u> the rain telling us he's fine? I know that sounds crazy or at least more like a Native American view. . . .

—CR

*   *   *

It is important to me to make regular visits to the cemetery, yet so painful. Those dates on the stone marking his grave are so stark, so harsh; announcing the facts of a too short life that has come and gone.

I know he is not there, that what we buried in that grave are only the ashes of that beautiful body. At the same time, he did live here and it seems essential to have a place denoting and honoring his presence, however brief, in this life, in this reality.

But even as I stand at his grave, I am aware of his presence in another reality. He is with me in so many ways, has let me know that the essential part of him continues on. He has come to me in dreams, has sent me messages in so many crazy and fun forms, has let me know that he is happy and well, has sent me his love. And I truly believe that our connection remains as deep as ever. I even believe we will be together again in this or another reality. But I can't help but wonder where he is now. His presence is so elusive, he seems so close and yet so far away.

What is this other level of reality in which I envision him now, or where is it? What does he do there? What is his "life" like now? How does he look? Has he aged? How can I learn more about where he is? How can I learn to see through the "veil" that separates our realities? Am I being greedy to want more?

—DSB

*   *   *

Strange how life in dreams is so much more real than life in reality, even after three years of this reality.

—LVR

*   *   *

When I lost my child, I lost my fear of death. I am not ready to leave yet but when the time comes, I don't think I will be afraid. If anything frightens me now it is the thought of having to leave those whom I love here. But I am mostly curious about what lies on the other side of this life.

—DSB

*   *   *

For as far back as I can remember, my father always said he would live until he was 85. Just weeks before his 85th birthday, he was diagnosed with a terminal illness. The doctors gave him 6 months to 2 years. Six months later he was gone.

When I was told that the end was near, my first reaction was strange but peaceful. I thought, "Well, here we go again." It was as though we had parted from each other in this way many times before.

Perhaps we have a knowing; we know more than we know we know. . . .

—DSB

*   *   *

Sometimes I wonder
is this where you've gone
Above clouds
pillow white
I look down and wonder
Do you live here now
Do you live somewhere else
Do you live.
In the clouds I am overcome
with thoughts of you.
Puffs of air
resting on top of the sky.
Stretching their billowy blanket
into the distance.
In this sky
I search
for signs
of you.

I sit above this world
and see so much more
than I ever did.
I turn my gaze down
and find a sunset.
This sunset
is a picture you
painted
high above
those who think they know,
yet who have never
themselves
truly watched
a setting sun.

—LVR

What is death in terms of what lies ahead for those who have died? Where do we go and how much awareness do we have of the life we have left behind? Do we continue to exist in some form or manner, or is this all there is? Certainly these are questions that plague the minds of those whose loved ones have died. Ultimately, each of us also is faced with similar kinds of questions as we seek to come to terms with our own mortality.

Although we cannot truly ever know the answers to such questions, interpretations in response to queries about what happens after death may be placed on a continuum ranging, at one end, from a belief in a state of nothingness or total annihilation to, at the other end, a perception that what occurs is a shift in reality which is part of an ongoing cycle of life, death, and rebirth. In between lie many notions about what death holds in store for each of us. These include beliefs in concepts such as heaven, hell, purgatory, and nirvana, to name but a few currently accepted in our society. What is more, "Belief in the immortality of the soul seems to be common to all religions and to the mythologies of various cultures" (Achte, 1980, p. 12). The various common interpretations of death which emerge from a spiritual perspective have been summarized as follows: "(1) a more enfeebled form of life, (2) the continuation of personal existence more or less as usual, (3) perpetual spiritual development, (4) a triphasic progression from waiting to judgment and on to a final eternal culmination (the most traditional form of Christian belief), (5) cycling and recycling of the self through life-death-rebirth passages, and (6) nothing" (Kastenbaum, 1986, p. 34).

The study of death-related traditions in many societies, both ancient and modern, reveals a further variety of viewpoints. For example, the process of mummification in ancient Egypt as well as in Peru indicates a strong belief in an afterlife in these societies. Similarly, the worldwide practice of including in the grave such practical items as food, drink, and tools speaks to earlier perceptions regarding life after death (Toynbee, 1980).

At the same time, Hindus—both ancient and modern—share a belief in an immortality described as "suprapersonal." In other words, there is an assumption that the essence of a human being's psyche is merged with ultimate reality after death. Buddhists, on the other hand, believe in an immortality described as "depersonalized." In this case, release from self-centeredness is the means by which one moves beyond or extinguishes the sense of the personal self manifested in a particular lifetime (Toynbee, 1980).

In recent years, study of the near-death experience has been the major focus of a number of researchers (Moody, 1977; Morse, 1990; Ring, 1984), and reports based on these studies continue to raise some interesting questions. Various accounts have revealed a pattern of similar events experienced by those who have returned to life after having been determined to be clinically dead. For example, most survivors report a sense of serenity and joy, of being welcomed on the other side by loving beings and of the presence of great light. And most also report the complete loss of their fear of death. Currently, the media—movies, books, TV—are saturated with stories related to the near-death experience, which may explain, or is at least coincident with, an increased willingness in our society to deal with the realm of death and dying.

Finally, it is also important to note that over the centuries and in various forms, volumes have been written in an attempt to understand and resolve the conundrum of death. According to the poet Richard Eberhart (in Packard, 1981), "Death is a final mystery. Birth is a mystery too—the deep question of why we were born as we are, beyond the know[n] physicality" (pp. xiv–xv). It is Eberhart's belief, however, that through the millennia, the poems that have been written about birth are not nearly as frequent or as deep as those whose subject is death. And once again, a multitude of perspectives related to the experience of death is revealed through a reading of these death-related poems.

As we reflect on the range of possible perspectives about death, and having considered the questions regarding the formation of our beliefs posed in the previous chapter, perhaps we have a sense of where we would be on a continuum of interpretive frameworks. Ideally, such a process of reflection has been informative for each of us personally and also has helped to underline the dilemma encountered when we attempt to define or describe what is meant by death. To be sure, one of the only things about which we may be certain is that death constitutes the end of life as we know it in this physical reality. What lies on the other side of death, however, remains an enigma.

By contrast, we know a great deal about dying and bereavement, both of which are available for examination and firsthand experience in ways that death is not. Nevertheless, the unknowable dimension of death often complicates both the process of dying, particularly for those whose life may be ending, and the experience of bereavement for those who survive. In addition, recent advances in technology which have increased dramatically the ability to sustain life also have led to enormous complexity related to all facets of death, dying, and bereavement.

This chapter explores some of the factors that may influence the ways in which different individuals understand and therefore react to death. It also looks more closely at the experience of dying as well as at some approaches to facilitating this process. The chapter concludes by defining and considering the bereavement process and examining some of the many explanatory models that have been created to describe what survivors go through following the death of a loved one. This chapter also provides an overview of some ways in which the bereaved may be supported and their pain ameliorated in the initial stages of the grief process.

DEATH

As mentioned previously, despite our traditional reluctance, recent years have witnessed a growing respect for, as well as increased attention to, the topic of death and dying. This is particularly true in the professional arena. For example, specialists in the relatively new field of thanatology now focus primarily on understanding and providing comfort to those who are dying. The hospice movement, whose goal is to help people die well (Byock, 1997), has evolved and has become an important component of service options for the dying. Furthermore, a variety of journals devote themselves solely to the publication of research and theory related to greater understanding of death and dying. At the societal level, increasingly we find discussions of death-related issues permeating the popular press. Particularly salient in this regard are controversies over the issues of abortion and euthanasia. These trends, evident both in the professional arena and among the general public, seem to be indicative of a greater willingness to accept, explore, and attempt to understand the meaning of life and its logical complement, death.

Despite this apparent shift in social attitudes and awareness, we nevertheless must remain sensitive to the unique ways in which individuals in a given context experience the phenomenon of death. Conversations about death still may remain difficult for many, including those whose lives are rapidly ending. What is more, even when conversation is possible, it is important to recognize that there are many influences on the creation of meaning for each person. Some of these influences include past experiences with death (Callanan & Kelley, 1992), family patterns related to loss and bereavement (Byng-Hall, 1991), stage in the family life cycle (McGoldrick & Walsh, 1991) and ethnic background (McGoldrick et al., 1991). The presence or absence of a religious or spiritual belief system also may be extremely significant. Another salient factor is that of the larger culture:

> Culture influences death concerns in virtually every way possible: it affects causes of death and the kinds of care that dying people receive; it influences perceptions of health caretakers and the methods used by health caretakers and who is entitled to be a health caretaker; it determines funeral rituals and burial rituals and whether remains are disposed of by earth, water, or fire; it has an effect on where the dying occurs, who is in attendance, and how the body is handled after death. It is impossible to exaggerate the role of culture. (Kalish, 1980, p. 46)

At the same time, it also is important to be aware that our concepts about death may shift and change over time. The following general propositions about our ideas of death (Shneidman, 1980a, p. 281), each of which is considered briefly, thus seem to be worthy of note. Included are the following:

1. The concept of death is always relative.
2. The concept of death is exceedingly complex.
3. Ideas about death change.
4. The developmental "goal" of death concepts is obscure, ambiguous, or still being evolved.
5. Death concepts are influenced by the situational context.
6. Death concepts are related to behavior.

In other words, an individual's thoughts about death emerge from and are influenced by the level of development currently attained by that person. Psychosocial, cognitive, and moral developmental stages, as well as chronological age, all have a bearing on our ability to create concepts in general. Certainly this applies as well to our ability to conceive of and formulate a belief system about death.

That the concept of death is complex reminds us that explanations generally take the form of groups of ideas rather than a single construct. In other words, each person has her or his story, or personal narrative, about death that may or may not be entirely coherent and is unlikely to be able to be articulated simply. Thus, both listening to and accurately interpreting a person's story about death also may involve a complex process requiring sensitivity, patience, and empathic understanding.

Given the notion that concepts about death are created relative to

developmental stages, and that all individuals grow and change, it is logical to assume that death-related concepts also will evolve and change
over time. Significant in this regard is the fact that each new experience
tends either to undermine or to validate to some extent our basic beliefs.
It is therefore understandable not only that concepts change but that they
may be insufficient or seriously challenged in times of crisis.

In addition, as we embrace a developmental perspective, we tend to
think in terms of a goal, or of an appropriate outcome ideally to be attained at each stage. Whereas some form of quantitative measure of prog-
ress is therefore possible relative to, for example, cognitive development,
the same cannot be said for the development of death-related concepts.
There is no ideal of maturity to which we can subscribe in this realm. Nor
can we assume that concepts of death created in childhood are necessarily
less adequate than those adopted in later life, possibly in conformity with
more socially accepted ideas.

Also consistent with the idea that death concepts are relative is the
awareness that specific situations color our perceptions. As noted in the
preface, it is one thing to think about death as an abstract concept and
quite another to come face to face with one's own mortality or the loss of
someone close. Similarly, the reactions of others, or specific circumstances
such as time of day or night, or what else is happening in our world, may
variously influence our thoughts and feelings in a given moment.

Finally, how an individual thinks about death also may influence
that person's behavior, although the connection may not necessarily be
conscious. For example, fears about death may manifest themselves in relationship problems as an individual questions his or her life choices. Or
the approach of a birthday marking attainment of the same age as that at
which a parent died may trigger anxiety without awareness of either the
underlying fear or its association with the deceased.

The idea of death, therefore, is ambiguous in many ways and for a variety of reasons. What is more, although the fact of death and its defini-
tion may at first glance appear to be much more obvious, the issue of what
constitutes death also has become somewhat unclear. This is particularly
true as we have moved into an era characterized by sophisticated medical
technology (Becvar, 2000a).

Indeed, in the context of a greatly increased ability to prolong life by
means of various life-support systems, both the medical community and
the legal community have struggled, for example, to delineate the differences between a vegetative state and brain death (Iglesias, 1995). In response to this issue, a set of standards for determining that the brain has

reached a condition in which it is deemed to be irreversibly nonfunctional was formulated in 1968 by a group of physicians at the Harvard Medical School. Now known as the Harvard Criteria, the presence of the following characteristics are understood to be indicators that death has occurred:

1. *Unreceptive and unresponsive.* No awareness is shown for external stimuli or inner need. The unresponsiveness is complete even under the application of stimuli that ordinarily would be extremely painful.
2. *No movements and no breathing.* There is a complete absence of spontaneous respiration and all other spontaneous muscular movement.
3. *No reflexes.* The usual reflexes that can be elicited in a neurophysiological examination are absent (e.g., when a light is shined in the eye, the pupil does not constrict).
4. *A flat EEG.* Electrodes attached to the scalp elicit a printout of electrical activity from the living brain. These are popularly known as *brain waves.* The respirator brain does not provide the usual pattern of peaks and valleys. Instead the moving automatic stylus records essentially a flat line. This is taken to demonstrate the lack of electrophysiological activity.
5. *No circulation to or within the brain.* Without the oxygen and nutrition provided to the brain by its blood supply, functioning will soon terminate. (Precisely how long the brain can retain its *viability,* the ability to survive, without circulation is a matter of much current investigation and varies somewhat with conditions.) (Kastenbaum, 1986, p. 9)

Over time, the Harvard Criteria have become the basis on which difficult decisions often are made. In addition, the field of bioethics, or biomedical ethics (Beauchamp & Childress, 1994), has been created in order to be able to respond appropriately to dilemmas at an institutional level. The goal is to facilitate the making of morally and ethically prudent decisions in the face of a biotechnology that has advanced to the point that the boundary between life and death often is blurred.

Nowhere, then, is the issue of death as unequivocal as we might wish or assume. We do not and cannot know what happens after we die and thus we must create theories or stories that satisfy our need to understand at some level. Our theories may or may not be adequate in times of crisis and we may find that the beliefs to which we subscribe are in conflict with those of others in our world. What is more, when the moment of death approaches, we often are faced with having to make decisions about what is life and what is death, when to unplug a machine, or how much suffering is appropriate. Thus, the process of dying also is often a complicated matter that demands of everyone involved far more than might have been anticipated, particularly as we place current concerns in historical context.

DYING

That is, there was a time in the not so distant past when living and dying were much simpler matters than they seem to have become in recent years, particularly in Western society. When people grew old and/or became seriously ill, there was little to be done except to make them as comfortable as possible and allow them to die. Today, however, we are both blessed and cursed by a remarkable ability to cure disease and to extend life even in the face of seriously debilitating terminal illnesses. Organ donation and transplantation, as well as the creation of a host of elaborate life-support systems, have played a particularly significant role in this regard. At the same time, the capacity to sustain life, often beyond the point of meaningful existence, also has spawned great controversy and conflict.

In fact, the need for an institutional response such as the field of bioethics represents has emerged in part in response to disputes regarding the manner of our death and the issue of who is to have control over our dying (Carter, 1996). Thus, for example, we are faced with questions such as the following: Are the decisions about the way the transition from life to death is going to occur to be left in the hands of the dying person or is it the families and communities of the dying that have responsibility for such decisions?

Those who have been instrumental in the development and support of the hospice movement in this country (Byock, 1997; Callanan & Kelley, 1992) believe the most appropriate response to terminal illness and the questions it raises is to provide supportive, palliative—rather than curative—care until physical death has been medically determined. By contrast, there are others who believe the option to hasten the dying process through some form of euthanasia should be available to persons who have determined that a reasonable quality of life has ceased (Battin, 1994; Dying Well Network, 1996). Ironically, the goal of facilitating a good death is shared by both groups, despite the fact that the means to this end certainly differ dramatically (Becvar, 2000a).

However, before a person with a terminal illness reaches the final phase of the dying process, when issues such as the foregoing are most likely to come into play, the person first must come to terms with the fact that death is imminent. According to the model developed by Elisabeth Kübler-Ross (1969), there are five stages that people tend to experience as life is ending. The first stage is distinguished by denial, when the person is unable or unwilling to accept the fact that she or he is dying. Rage and anger, or resentment about the fact that one's life is coming to an end, characterize the second stage. In the third, or bargaining stage, the person attempts to gain more time by, for example, promising God that he or she will be a better person or will engage in more humanitarian behavior. As the person moves into the fourth stage and acknowledges the inevitable, depression, or grief and sadness, may be felt in response to the fact that death is imminent. The fifth and final stage is acceptance, or at least a feeling of resignation, as the person recognizes that his or her life is indeed nearly over.

While such a model certainly is not invariant for every person, nor are the stages necessarily followed in the sequence described, familiarity with the model may assist support persons in understanding the behavior of an individual at various points in the dying process. At the same time, however, we also must be aware that a dying person may have little or no trouble accepting and coming to terms with the fact of his or her dying. Thus, it is important to remain cognizant of the fact that, as Ira Byock (1997) notes, "the actual range of human experience of dying is broad" (p. xiv).

For some, including Kübler-Ross (1975), the dying process also may be perceived and engaged in as a final stage of growth, one that is understood as a transformative experience (Callanan & Kelley, 1992). This kind of perspective is consistent with the Buddhist belief that "when we accept death, transform our attitude toward life, and discover the fundamental connection between life and death, a dramatic possibility for healing can occur" (Sogyal, 1992, p. 31).

Espousing a similar perspective, Anya Foos-Graber (1989), a student of Eastern philosophy, uses the term "deathing" to describe a focus on actively and consciously engaging in one's own dying in order to facilitate the growth of one's innermost being, or the soul. She sees the deathing process, which she compares to the birthing process, as "a means of making an informed, safe, responsible, and joyous transition from the physically focused 'I' consciousness to the various subtle stages of life-after-death's expanded states, including humanity's birthright—full enlightenment, or liberation" (p. 200).

The deathing process, or conscious dying, as described by Foos-

Graber (1989) involves the use of a variety of breathing techniques and meditative practices. According to this perspective, dying thus is understood as one aspect of a larger spiritual discipline, or art form, one that facilitates transformation to higher states of consciousness. In contrast to the view that death is just one more biological process which simply happens to us, the person who is dying is encouraged to become an active participant, to embrace death and to use the experience in as growthful a manner as possible.

Although one may find it difficult to accept fully a perspective such as that offered by deathing, the idea of seeing death as a stage of growth not unlike other developmental phases may prove helpful to those faced with terminal illness. Despite the fact that having foreknowledge about the timing of one's death may be frightening, at least at first, it may provide an opportunity to make the best use of the time remaining. Certainly it may prove helpful as well for those who survive to have been active and supportive participants in a meaningful dying process.

In this regard, hospice nurses Maggie Callanan and Patricia Kelley (1992) believe that those who are caring for the dying should be aware of the many aspects of "nearing death awareness." For example, they report that a common occurrence among the terminally ill is the experience of visions. These visions may include a sense of the presence of departed loved ones, of spiritual beings, of a bright light, or of being in a particular place. Those who are dying also may report that they have felt great warmth and love, not unlike the accounts of those who have had a near-death experience.

Engaging in a life review also is often a typical experience among those who are dying. And although there may be a variety of reactions to this process, it is interesting to note that those near death generally do not report feeling fear as the end approaches. Rather, their greatest concerns tend to be about those who will be left behind. Indeed, it is not unusual for children to send their parents away just prior to their death, whether to protect their parents and/or to enable themselves to complete their dying. What is more, dying people generally seem to prefer to die at home if this is at all possible. And the families of the dying prefer truthful reports about diagnosis, prognosis, and what to expect.

In all cases, according to Callanan and Kelley (1992), close observation of the dying reveals awareness of the communication of important messages to family, friends, and other caregivers. Although sometimes difficult to decipher because they may be in the form of symbols or metaphors, these messages may be sorted into two categories:

The first category of messages described what patients were experiencing: being in the presence of someone not alive, the need to prepare for travel or a change, mentions of some place they alone could see, their knowledge of when death would occur.

The second category consisted of messages about something, or someone, needed so death could be peaceful: the desire to reconcile personal, spiritual, or moral relationships, and requests to remove some barrier to achieving this peace. (Callanan & Kelley, 1992, pp. 29–30)

It therefore becomes very important for caregivers to learn how to listen well and to try to understand what the dying person is attempting to express. Being able to respond appropriately certainly may facilitate a more comfortable death for the dying person. In addition, it also may provide a measure of comfort as well as a sense of meaning and resolution for those who survive.

Byock (1997) adds the notions that we do not necessarily die as we have lived and that there is a great potential for personal growth in the dying process. Indeed, he notes that an important aspect of dying is what is called by hospice " 'the five things of relationship completion'—saying 'I forgive you'; 'Forgive me', Thank you'; 'I love you'; and 'Goodbye' " (Byock, 1997, p. 140). He suggests that as caregivers are able to recognize requests for assistance, the sting of death may be somewhat alleviated.

Thus, although both having a loved one die and being intimately involved in the details and demands of caregiving may be challenging for everyone involved, the experience also is one that has great potential to create healing: "The decisions people make to complete their dying days, or to help someone they love complete a life, are rarely easy. They are often gut-wrenching and may challenge basic beliefs about who one is and what is important. Nevertheless, these end-of-life decisions create opportunities for new experiences and discoveries that range from the fairly mundane to the frankly extraordinary" (Byock, 1997, p. 137).

There are thus several facets of the dying process about which it would seem appropriate to be sensitive. Choosing to allow family members to care for oneself as death approaches may be an act of great love. Choosing to care for a beloved dying person also may be an act of great love. Enabling the dying person to resolve relationship issues and to continue to grow until her or his last breath is taken communicates far more than words may express. Responding appropriately to the final needs of the dying person demonstrates caring and sensitivity and enables the caregiver to feel a sense of purpose. And having been able to participate in a meaningful way may help to ease the inevitable pain that follows the death of a loved one. That is, the intensity of the bereavement process may be, at least in part, a reflection of the experience of the dying process.

BEREAVEMENT

Whether death is feared or embraced, and regardless of the manner of dying, those who survive are faced with the task of coping with the loss, the process known as bereavement. According to Kastenbaum (1986), grief is one response to the experience of bereavement whereas mourning may be understood as "the culturally patterned expression of the bereaved person's thoughts and feelings" (p. 139). In our society many of the typical expressions of grief include feelings of confusion and despair, forgetfulness, sleep disturbances, and extended periods of crying, as well as a variety of physical symptoms. These responses are certainly to be expected, and therefore typically are accepted as normal, but what is considered to be the appropriate degree of intensity and duration also is socially prescribed and has been the subject of much debate through the years.

Classical models of the grieving process were based on the psychoanalytic perspectives of Freud (1917/1957) and Lindemann (1944) as well as on the attachment theory of Bowlby (1980). Until quite recently, most professional explanations were derived from their work. Based on such models, it was understood that all important relationships involve an investment of energy. Thus, when a person dies, it was assumed that the survivor must withdraw the energy previously invested in the relationship with the deceased in order that he or she might be able to form new attachments. The inability to complete this process of energy withdrawal in an appropriate and timely manner was indicative of problems and even of pathology.

According to these classical models it also was assumed that the grieving process is time-limited (Peretz, 1970), with the standard being 2 weeks during which the survivor experienced shock and intense grief. These first 2 weeks were then followed by 2 months of strong grieving. And finally, there were 2 years during which the grief decreased, the bereaved individual recovered, and she or he returned to full, normal functioning. By the end of this 2-year period the grieving process was to have concluded. Throughout the grieving process, the basic goal was that of detaching from emotional ties to the deceased in order to be able to form new relationships with those who were still living (Bowlby, 1980). Finally, should the grief not be resolved within the designated appropriate amount of time, mourning was to be considered maladaptive (Raphael, 1983).

Such an approach not only was subscribed to for many years follow-ing its creation but also continues today to remain influential in the work and thinking of many clinicians (Nolen-Hoeksma & Larson, 1999). How-ever, during the 1980s a variety of studies challenged all three of its funda-mental assumptions (Demi & Miles, 1987; Fish, 1986; Fulton, 1987; Knapp, 1987; McClowry, Davies, May, Kulenkamp, & Martinson, 1987; Osterweis, Solomon, & Green, 1984; Palmer, 1987; Zisook & Schucter, 1986), which may be summarized as follows: "(a) bereaved people go through predictable stages of grief; (b) depression following loss is inevita-ble, and people who do not experience severe distress over the loss will eventually show some psychopathology, and (c) working through the loss is essential to recovery" (Nolen-Hoeksma & Larson, 1999, p. 15).

By contrast, based on the findings reported in the more recent stud-ies, as well as on current research in the area of stress and coping, bereave-ment began to be looked at in context, with consideration given to the impact on the bereavement process of individual beliefs and coping skills. Given this shift in perspective, new conclusions were formulated. First, it was recognized that the grieving process may have no fixed end point, and, indeed, that it may last a lifetime. Although the bereaved person may return to normal functioning, she or he may never "get over" the loss but, rather, is faced with the challenge of learning to live with it.

Second, complete detachment from the deceased came to be under-stood as neither desirable nor possible. In other words, there is now recog-nition that the bereaved person is able to maintain a simultaneous attach-ment to both the living and to the one who has died and still function perfectly well. For example, according to one paradigm (Silverman & Klass, 1996), it is understood that "interdependence is sustained even in the absence of one of the parties . . . . the bereaved remain involved and connected to the deceased, and . . . actively construct an inner represen-tation of the deceased that is part of the normal grieving process" (p. 16).

Finally, an awareness emerged that bereavement may take many forms and that the degree to which it is adaptive or maladaptive can only be determined on an individual basis. From the perspective of stress and coping models (Nolen-Hoeksma & Larson, 1999), acknowledgment also was given to the tremendous challenge to belief systems, to daily life, and to the self-concept that the loss of someone close represents. It therefore follows that the need to reorganize on all three of these fronts is an inevi-table aspect of bereavement. Indeed, according to thanatologist Therese

Rando (1997), acute grief responses share similarities with those of post-traumatic stress disorder and include the necessity for the following:

> the working through of related affects, integration of conscious and dissoci-
> ated aspects, mourning of relevant secondary physical and psychosocial
> losses, acquisition of new ways of being to move adaptively into the new
> world, development of a comprehensive perspective on the event and one's
> level of control therein, emotional relocation of what was lost, acceptance
> of fitting responsibility and relinquishment of inappropriate guilt, revisions
> of the assumptive world demanded by the event and its repercussions, cre-
> ation of meaning out of the experience, integration of the event into the to-
> tality of one's life, formation of a new identity reflecting survival of the
> event, and appropriate reinvestment in life. (p. xvii)

Finally, based on recent research studies, professionals now recognize that the process of coming to terms with one's grief is particularly difficult either when the circumstances of the death represent a threat to one's worldview, especially one's basic beliefs about such issues as goodness or justice in the world, or when little social support is evidenced. Further, those whose coping styles involve either avoidance or excessive rumination may have more difficulty dealing with bereavement. And people who tend to be dependent, to be pessimistic, and to lack self-control and/or who are emotionally less stable also are likely to experience greater difficulty making the adjustments required (Nolen-Hoeksma & Larson, 1999).

The shift in perspective represented by the more recent models of bereavement reminds us that rather than pathologizing an individual's grief process, what we are called on to do is to understand each person's reactions in the context of his or her worldview and unique situation. Further, according to such a perspective, the goal becomes one of facilitating adaptation (J. K. Bernstein, 1997) rather than one of overcoming and recovering from a major loss. There is simultaneously acknowledgment that given the nature of this process, one's values, attitudes, beliefs, perceptions, and relationships will all be affected and altered and one will be forever changed as a function of the experience.

Given the enormity of the task involved as the bereaved face the challenge of dealing with their pain and searching for answers to their questions, we must recognize the variety of reactions and range of emotions that may accompany their grief and sadness. Some of these reactions and emotions include confusion about the presumed injustice of the death, a sense of desperation and tremendous anger, the latter often directed at God, especially when no solace seems to be forthcoming from this resource. As theologian C. S. Lewis (1976) queries in the well-known book *A Grief Observed*, written shortly after the death of his beloved wife:

> Meanwhile, where is God? This is one of the most disquieting symptoms. When you are happy, so happy that you have no sense of needing Him, so happy that you are tempted to feel His claims upon you as an interruption, if you remember yourself and turn to Him with gratitude and praise, you will be—or so it feels—welcomed with open arms. But go to Him when your need is desperate, when all other help is vain, and what do you find? A door slammed in your face, and a sound of bolting and double bolting on the inside. After that, silence. You may as well turn away. The longer you wait, the more emphatic the silence will become. There are no lights in the windows. It might be an empty house. Was it ever inhabited? It seemed so once. And that seeming was as strong as this. What can this mean? Why is He so present a commander in our time of prosperity and so very absent a help in time of trouble? (pp. 4–5)

Indeed, Lewis's story provides a useful illustration of several important facets of the bereavement process: Despite a deep faith characterized by a strong belief in God, his entire worldview was called into question as he attempted to make sense of and reconcile himself to his wife's death. And although ultimately he was able to regain his faith, he nevertheless was unable to get over his loss. Finally, although he continued to pursue an active and productive career, his stepson (Gresham, 1988) reports that he became a different person from the one he had been while his wife was alive.

At the same time, and as a function of the assault to their worldview that may occur, as well as of the ensuing sense of uncertainty and confusion that may be experienced, those going through the bereavement process may evidence a much greater willingness than previously was the case to explore a variety of new and different viewpoints. This openness may be problematic for others, but it also can be a great resource if understood and accessed appropriately. The key for those who are attempting to support the bereaved is to be open themselves and aware of the potential utility of broad exploration.

For example, just as the dying may report what they consider to be valid encounters with departed loved ones, as well as a variety of other paranormal experiences, the bereaved may find themselves drawn to investigate psychic phenomena. Such investigations may be part of a search for reassurance about the well-being of the persons who have died and/or they may be undertaken in order to find answers to questions for which no logical responses seem able to be found. However, even while actively pursuing such avenues, there may be a sense on the part of the bereaved that they are going crazy as they get involved in such an arena, and this behavior may not fit with previous and perhaps long-held beliefs about themselves. They therefore may be unwilling even to discuss their activities and may thus deprive themselves of the reassurance of knowing that many others, who also are far from crazy, have followed a similar path.

To explain, there currently appear to be more and more books written about communications with departed loved ones as well as about the comfort and hope provided by such communications (cf. Anderson & Barone, 2000; Martin & Romanowski, 1994; Van Praagh, 2000). And given our inability to know what happens after death, we must not be too hasty to condemn or invalidate pursuits in this area. Rather, what appears to be crucial is guidance and support focused on ensuring that whatever resources the bereaved choose to avail themselves of have a reputation for credibility and ethical behavior. We also must respect and affirm the ability of those with whom we are working to trust their own innate wisdom about appropriate choices.

Also significant in this regard is the fact that receiving comfort and perhaps hopefulness about the possibility that life and relationships continue even after death usually does not take away the grief experienced as a function of the loss. It certainly may be reassuring to know that our loved ones continue to exist in spirit form or are happy, or that one day we may be together again. Nevertheless, the loss of their physical presence, the void in our lives, continues to be real and is certainly likely to remain even in the face of such reassurance.

Another area of pursuit that may be helpful for the bereaved, one that certainly may be perceived as less threatening to everyone involved, is to read about the experiences of others who have walked a similar path. For example, there are a variety of books written by parents who have lost children (J. R. Bernstein, 1997; J. Bernstein, 2000; Bramblett, 1991; Claypool, 1974; Schiff, 1977; Wolterstorff, 1987); children who have lost parents (Brooks, 1999; Edelman, 1994); and spouses who have lost wives or husbands (Lewis, 1976; Van Auken, 1977). Many more resources also are available which focus on specific types of death not only within each of the categories mentioned but also within many others. These books may provide valuable information for there seems to be a measure of comfort to be found in learning that what one is experiencing is not unlike the reports of others who have been faced with similar kinds of loss.

Indeed, the need to focus on specific kinds of loss, as well as helpful responses within each category, brings us to the conclusion of this chapter. However, in the next eight chapters I pick up this train of thought as we consider the variety of ways in which death may occur. And a crucial aspect of the discussions in each of these chapters is the ramifications for the bereaved as well as various ways we may be supportive in the presence of their grief.

THERAPEUTIC CONVERSATIONS
AND REFLECTIONS

∾

The wife and husband who sat facing me on the couch in my therapy room were obviously deeply distressed. They took turns telling their tale, the one filling in for the other when tears prevented either from speaking further. They described a beautiful daughter, the oldest of five children, who had attended college in another state. They spoke of intense struggles over the years but of finally having become close as their daughter achieved success in her studies, chose a career that was important to her, and created meaningful relationships with roommates and friends. They had been so relieved to get beyond the fears that clouded the stormy period of her early adolescence. Now, all their hopes and dreams had been shattered by her death under unclear circumstances.

While away at school, their daughter had come home late one night from a party to which she had gone with several friends. Although she was reported to have had one or two drinks, she was not intoxicated. She apparently also had not used drugs of any kind. In the morning, however, when her roommates tried to awaken her, she was dead. An autopsy had been performed and a poisonous chemical had been found to be the cause of death. Still to be decided was whether the chemical had been ingested accidentally or had been given to her by someone else, or whether she had ended her own life.

The parents had brought their daughter's body home, where

they had been able to have the funeral and burial services. Although there had been a great deal of publicity in the local newspapers, their friends and family members had been supportive. No one, particularly her siblings, could believe that she had committed suicide, and all who knew her were horrified both by her death and by the uncertainty surrounding it.

The parents were convinced that although there might have been a time when their daughter could have taken her own life, this just could not be the case now. They knew she would have had familiarity with and access to the chemical because of the classes she was taking. But they also were aware of how happy she had become. Classmates who also could have had access to the chemical were being questioned because of the possibility of foul play. However, no one believed that someone could have killed the young woman intentionally. At the same time, everyone was confused about how she could have gotten the chemical into her system accidentally.

In addition to their grief, the parents were assailed by doubts and questions. Nevertheless, they were going to have to await the official ruling following a hearing that was to be held 2 weeks later. To add to their stress, they would have to travel back to the other state to attend the hearing. What is more, they were extremely anxious that the official ruling might not fit their own convictions.

That is, although they did not know what had happened, one of their other children had had a dream about their daughter in which she gave an assurance that she was fine and that she had not taken her own life. Both parents were holding firmly to this belief and were simply confused about the other two possibilities. In an effort to find some answers, both parents had been exploring the Internet, looking for psychics who might be able to assist them. They were reticent to share with me either the dream or their activities relative to psychics, but I let them know that many parents found both kinds of explorations to be extremely reassuring. Moreover, I was able to refer them to someone in this realm whom I knew to be reputable.

After discussing other ways in which the parents could begin the process of healing, both for themselves and their other children, we agreed to meet again once they had had a chance to follow up with the referral. They returned about 3 weeks later, feeling some-
(cont.)

what better. Prior to the hearing, they had gotten a reading in which, once again, their daughter had assured her parents that she had not taken her own life. She also sent messages of love and gratitude to them and to her siblings in a way that enabled the parents to believe they truly were communicating with their daughter. They then attended the hearing and received a decision that left the circumstances undetermined. They were truly relieved that it had not been judged either a murder or a suicide. Although they knew they would wonder forever what had happened, they felt that an enormous weight had been lifted.

Clearly, this is only the beginning of their story. However, it is for me one of the most crucial parts. To explain, I became aware quickly that the parents wanted and needed validation for their pursuits in the realms of dreams and psychics. I also recognized how fearful they were that I would perceive them as crazy. And I was concerned that whomever they met with be ethical and not do anything to hurt them further. Fortunately, because of my own explorations, I am able to share my experiences with similar activities as well as the ways in which I believe it is safest to pursue them. I also am able to make referrals to people I know personally and whose work I trust. Indeed, with the parents' agreement, we all were able to work together to facilitate the meeting which the parents ultimately found to be so helpful.

CHAPTER 3

When Death Comes Unannounced

◇

It has been years since my son's death, and yet the horror of those first few hours remains.

It began with a Saturday afternoon phone call, a female voice asking if my son was there. I said no. She then gave me her name, told me she was a nurse, said she was calling from the hospital. I went cold all over as she reported that there had been an accident, that they had taken "lots and lots" of X rays, that I needed to come. She had to repeat directions to the hospital several times before I could take them in.

I raced down to my husband's office in the basement, telling him my son had been in an accident, we had to go to the hospital. We fairly flew out the front door, calling to the young man who was painting our house that my son was hurt, asking him to lock up when he left.

The ride to the hospital was nightmarish. I was so frightened, so cold.

The nurse, waiting for us in the emergency room, said my son was in surgery.

The doctors were noncommittal, wanted permissions. I said do what you need to do, just save my son.

The other boy had been seriously injured, but he would be OK.

I called my daughter, had a co-worker bring her to the hospital. Told her what had happened.

With help from a kindly long-distance operator I was able to locate my son's father, told him what had happened, that he better come.

The police wanted to talk with us, said it had been an accident. Said the driver of the car had "cheated" a little over the yellow line. Said the driver had been a paramedic, was responsible for resuscitating my son, had gotten his wife to go for help.

He had been taken to the hospital by helicopter. Said it had taken several *hours to locate me because we had different last names. They hadn't checked the pouch on his bicycle where his identification information was kept.*

I called my parents, told them what had happened, said we would not be visiting them this week as planned. Asked them to activate their prayer network.

I left a message for the rector of our church, described briefly what had happened, where we were.

Friends—ours, my son's, my daughter's—began arriving, and the long vigil began. We were moved from one waiting room to another. There were hours with no information. Eventually most went home, although a few of those closest to us remained.

My son's employers, both physicians, arrived. They had seen him. They were able to explain what was going on, told us how serious things were, tried to prepare us for what we would see when we were allowed to visit him.

He was unconscious. He was not recognizable as the handsome healthy young man who had left that morning to swim, ride his bike, and then run as he continued his triathlon training. But I knew him nevertheless. Knew the body that he had shaved to gain speed. Knew the beautiful and beloved person he was despite the incredible disfigurement.

We sat with him as long as we were allowed. We talked to him, told him how much we loved him, begged him to get well.

When we left his room, I was overcome by dizziness, almost fainted, had to lie on the floor in the hallway until I had regained my equilibrium.

My son's father arrived after what was for him a bitter and seemingly endless trip as he traveled from several states away.

The long night continued. I was so cold. My stomach hurt. A friend did some healing touch. I kept asking about my daughter, was she OK?

A chaplain came. Different religion—which bothered him more than us—and we welcomed his prayers.

We were allowed several more brief visits. There were tubes and machines everywhere with a nurse constantly monitoring and charting. At one point things began to look more hopeful. Perhaps he was going to make it after all, despite the severity of his injuries.

Very early Sunday morning, our Episcopal priest arrived. Said he had been out of town, had just returned. Told us he had visited my son, had anointed him. Prayed with us, said he would offer prayers for him in church that morning.

We forced ourselves to eat some breakfast. The only thing I could manage was toast—it tasted like cardboard.

Things began to look worse. The doctor talked to us about turning off the respirator. Said we all have to die sometime—not a good remark to the mother of a 22-year-old. Said they would like to do a brain scan.

A social worker arrived, talked with us about the possibility of organ dona-
tion, explained the procedure. A gentle man who did a hard job well.

More waiting, wondering, praying.

The results of the brain scan indicated no hope. Our psychic friend said
that death probably had occurred in the predawn hours.

We decided to donate his kidneys. His body was maintained on a respirator
until after the surgery was completed.

Then we were allowed our final visit.

We gathered around his bed, holding each other, touching him, telling him
again how much we loved him. After 26 hours of waiting and hoping, we had to
say our good-byes.

Friends drove us home. I was still so cold.

The tears that until then had not been shed began; they continue to this
day. No longer as many or as often, but still they come. I expect they always
will each time I dare to relive this experience.

As I think back I remember that so many worries plagued me. Did he expe-
rience pain? Did he know what was happening? Did he know how much we
loved him? Did he get enough dinner the night before the accident? Why hadn't I
spent more time with him that morning before he left?

I also had so many unanswerable questions. How could this happen? What
did we do wrong? Where was the justice? We were all good people, trying to live
good lives. We had been on top of the world, new jobs, new lives beginning.
Both children were incredible—the fulfillment of every parent's dream. He and
his sister adored each other, reconnecting now as young adults. He was bursting
with life and plans. And now, suddenly, he was gone forever.

And we had so much to deal with. We wanted cremation, but it had to
wait. Accidental death in our state meant a mandatory autopsy.

The newspaper misspelled his name in the death notices. A phone call led
to a front-page headline after the story was told. Harassment of cyclists a "hot"
issue.

Family, friends, food all arriving. Phone ringing constantly. Cards pouring
in.

Met with a lawyer to discuss possible indictment of the driver by a grand
jury. Also possible lawsuits.

His college roommate appeared on our doorstep. He had thrown some
things into a paper bag, gotten on a plane and come to be with us. Just sat at the
bottom of the stairs and stared into space. Couldn't comprehend what had hap-
pened.

Met with our priest. Went to a funeral home. Wrote an obituary. Chose
the casket for the cremation. Knew immediately that the vigil and memorial ser-
vice would be held at our church.

Picked hymns: "The strife is o'er, the battle done, the victory of life is won"
had been running through my head from the time I woke up the first morning af-
ter. Also, "Amazing Grace," "And He Shall Feed His Flock."
    Found the poem: "To an Athlete Dying Young."
    Flowers for the altar—white roses and baby's breath. He was my baby.
    Beautiful, gut-wrenching ceremonies, wonderful tributes. Church crowded
to overflowing.
    My daughter magnificent as she read the poem she had written late the
night before the memorial service: "Let Me Run with You."
    One of our students described the whole experience as surreal.
    He was right.

—DSB

The distinguishing features in the case of sudden or accidental death are
the stresses and challenges to the coping ability of the bereaved (Rando,
1988). Survivors confront the pain of the loss at the same time that they
must deal with the shock, disbelief, and extreme disruption which suddenly are manifest in all areas of their lives. It is in such a state that they
must make decisions regarding essential issues such as organ donation, funeral preparations, and burial arrangements. In addition, they must contact family and friends, who also are shocked, and are faced with the necessity of recounting the details of what has happened over and over. And
they also must respond to the grief as well as to the daily needs of other
family members. All this takes place in a context in which there has been
no warning and, often, no prior preparation.

    What is most significant, however, is the challenge that is unique to
an unanticipated death. It involves the struggle to make sense of an event
that both occurred "out of the blue" and also may seem totally meaningless and incomprehensible. In one moment, one is transported from having a relationship with a person assumed to be perfectly normal and
healthy to having no relationship at all. What is more, the cause of death,
for example, when violence has been involved, may be particularly difficult to understand and accept (Nolen-Hoeksema & Larson, 1999). It is
not surprising, then, that in this case the grieving process may take longer
or be more complicated than in other instances of bereavement.

    Those who are bereaved in the aftermath of a death which has come
unannounced are likely to experience an overwhelming sense that suddenly they have no control, that the world has gone crazy. In addition, a
host of emotional manifestations that may run the gamut from numbness

to heartrending reactions and outbursts (Nurmi & Williams, 1997) are not at all uncommon. There also may be a greater tendency for the unexpectedly bereaved to experience physical symptoms. High blood pressure, colds and other infections, arthritis, chest pains, and allergies (Kastenbaum, 1986) often are evidenced in the aftermath of such a death. At the same time, however, it also is important to be aware that the ability of those who have encountered the sudden death of a loved one to adapt over the long term tends to be similar to that of those dealing with a death that was anticipated (J. R. Bernstein, 1997).

Facilitating such adaptation seems to require, above all, acknowledgment of the extent of the onslaught to the belief system of the bereaved that the experience of an unanticipated death usually represents. As noted in the previous chapter, all the fundamental assumptions that had been held dear may be destroyed in a single stroke. Hence the survivor is bereft on two counts. Not only is the loved one gone, but so also is one's worldview, or the means by which one previously had made sense of one's reality. As described in Chapter 1, such an experience is comparable to being set adrift, at sea, without compass or anchor, not knowing where to go or how to get there even if one had the vaguest idea about the proper direction.

Thus, in our efforts to help we must recognize the need of those so bereaved to be able to create a meaningful story, or context, within which to make sense of the death. Indeed, to be able to recommit to life, to figure out a direction as well as to acquire the tools that may enable us to begin heading there, the construction of a whole new set of beliefs may be required. The substance of this new worldview may be drawn both from old ideas and assumptions that continue to remain useful and meaningful as well as from a wide range of alternative perspectives.

Before proceeding with a consideration of the process of reconstructing worldviews, however, a variety of factors also may need to be figured into the helping equation. Some important questions requiring attention include the following: How did the person die? Who, if anyone, was responsible? If it was health related, was there some way the death could have been prevented? If the death occurred as the result of an accident, was it truly accidental? Was the person who died negligent in any way? Was it a violent or wrongful death? Was the death a suicide? Does the death fall into the category of ambiguous loss? How much involvement will there be on the part of the legal justice system? Was an autopsy required? Will there be an inquest and/or a trial?

Answers to each of these questions provide further information about both the nature of the experience and what will be entailed for everyone involved in the days and months ahead. Ultimately, the bereaved will need support throughout the process of coming to terms with the loss in a way that is sensitive to and appropriate given the unique aspects of the situation. Truly, "the circumstances of different types of losses may require different strategies for coping and different types of support from family members and friends" (Nolen-Hoeksema & Larson, 1999, p. 33).

Throughout such a process we also need to understand that the healing journey may require a great amount of time as well as much searching in a variety of directions before the bereaved regain a sense of peace. To provide a fuller sense of the issues and requirements likely to be involved during such a process, this chapter looks at some of the specific aspects of several of the ways in which unanticipated death may occur as well as at some of the ramifications of each. Consideration is given to death caused by physical problems, accidental death, violent or wrongful death, suicide, and ambiguous death and loss. Finally, the chapter concludes with some thoughts about the meaning of social support as well as ways to help the bereaved both mourn their loss and complete business that may have been left unfinished as a function of a death that has come unannounced.

DEATH CAUSED BY PHYSICAL PROBLEMS

Dying in one's sleep or "dropping dead" in the midst of normal activities as the result of a heart attack represent just two of the ways in which death may occur suddenly as a function of physical problems. Or perhaps death occurred following routine surgery, when the patient unexpectedly experienced a blood clot in the lungs or cardiac arrest. Equally distressing and further illustrative may be the case of the athlete who collapses and dies during a practice or competition due, for example, to a ruptured aneurysm or an undiagnosed heart defect. In all such instances, though the cause of death certainly may be determined, its unexpected nature may make it extremely traumatic for the survivors.

In addition to the bewilderment over the loss, what may be most troubling is the feeling that the death could have been prevented. There thus may be a tendency or a desire to assign blame to self or others. Perhaps a spouse may feel that she or he should have noticed symptoms along the way. Perhaps there were some warning signs that the person who died ignored, despite the urging of other family members to seek medical attention. Perhaps parents may feel that they were responsible given lack of knowledge about a condition that made a child more vulnerable. Perhaps there is a perception that there was negligence on the part of medical personnel or others in a position of authority.

Dealing with anger and guilt thus becomes an important part of the bereavement process when sudden death has occurred as a result of physical problems. Indeed, in this instance, knowing the cause of death may be a hindrance rather than a help. At the same time, some small consolation may be found in situations in which death came swiftly and was therefore painless. At least the agony of wondering whether the person who died suffered is avoided. As always, however, this mitigating factor is more or less meaningful depending on other considerations (e.g., age at time of death).

To explain, if an elderly person dies in his or her sleep, survivors may experience gratitude. In this case, although technically "sudden," there was awareness that death probably was not too far away. Survivors therefore may be comforted by the fact that a protracted illness was avoided and that the person was able to slip away easily and peacefully. By contrast, when it is the relatively young parent of two children who dies in his or her sleep, little solace may be provided by the fact that she or he did not suffer.

As always, except in a general way, we really cannot predict exactly how survivors will respond. In this as in every case of unanticipated death, the feelings of grief may be accompanied by a variety of emotional reactions in response to the particular set of circumstances surrounding the death. And certainly this also holds true when death occurs as the function of an accident.

ACCIDENTAL DEATH

Some synonyms for the word "accident" include chance, fluke, serendipity, luck, circumstance, and twist of fate. The word "accident" also connotes a mishap, a mistake, a blunder (McCutcheon, 1995). Thus, it is not uncommon in the case of accidental death for survivors to second-guess themselves, to perhaps feel guilty for not having done things differently, to see themselves as somehow involved in causing the fatality. We must be sensitive to the fact that "the most agonizing instances of self-reproach and self-blame are generated in cases of accidental death. Such accidents, which highlight and fix in time a particular sequence in the ordinary flow of events, typically create the impression that a particular act or sequence of acts caused the death even when this sense of cause and effect is illusory or misleading" (Shapiro, 1994, p. 264).

Therefore, when attempting to support those bereaved by an accidental death it is important to try to prevent self-blame that is neither logical nor justified. For example, the fact that the death of a teenager occurred at home while the parents were away on a trip certainly does not mean either that the parents should not have gone away or that somehow they were responsible for their child's death. Nor are the feelings of guilt deserved, especially when steps had been taken to ensure the well-being of the teenager. Nevertheless, parents in such a case certainly may be assailed by the thought that if they had stayed at home, if they had returned sooner, if, if, if, the death would not have occurred. All this may be true, but the fact that the parents were absent did not cause the death. What is more, we really don't have enough knowledge about how and why death occurs when it does to be able to deny that it might have happened anyway, although perhaps under slightly different circumstances and at a slightly different time.

On the other hand, when a true sense of responsibility and accountability is an appropriate response, it is important that it not be ignored or dealt with in too superficial a manner. If the course of events surrounding the death include misjudgment or carelessness, for example, speeding in a car or failing to observe traffic signals, feelings of remorse or regret on the part of the driver need to be allowed if not encouraged. Being able to own one's part in what has transpired allows for the opportunity to make amends, to deal with guilt that is logical in a way that is both healthy and meaningful for everyone involved. Thus the driver may learn to forgive her- or himself and thereby be able to go on with life in a more functional manner. In addition, the family of the person who has died may experience some alleviation of their anguish given the recognition of responsibility and expression of contrition on the part of the driver.

Indeed, what may be particularly difficult for survivors are situations in which there was clear responsibility on the part of another for the death of a loved one but no acknowledgment of this participation. And such situations may be further exacerbated when the legal system, on which one has relied for the meting out of justice, fails to support what appear to be the obvious facts of the situation. Thus, there is anger that someone who bears responsibility for the death of a loved one is unwilling or unable to acknowledge guilt. This anger may be exacerbated further when the system also seems to let us down. For the bereaved it is injustice piled on injustice and certainly is a significant complicating factor in the ability to heal. Not only is such a scenario true in the case of accidental death, but it may be even more significant in circumstances involving violent or wrongful death.

VIOLENT OR WRONGFUL DEATH

Certainly another whole dimension is added to the grieving process following sudden death when the loved one has been the victim of murder or has died as the result of some other form of violence. In this instance, it is typical for survivors to become obsessed with concerns that great suffering may have been experienced by the loved one in the process of dying (Knapp, 1987). Rage about the injustice of the situation (J. R. Bernstein, 1997) is also highly likely. As the legal justice system becomes involved, insult may be added to injury by the requirement for an autopsy, by delays in the handling of the case and/or by the ultimate lack of satisfactory resolution.

Another difficult aspect, which also may occur in the context of accidental death, is the likelihood of disfigurement or mutilation of the body of the person who has died. Thus, the bereaved person's final memory is an image that is not only appalling but often remains to haunt him or her long years later. This image adds to fears we may have about the degree of suffering and pain of which the loved one may have been aware. What is more, depending on the extent of the damage, the possibility of allowing the body to be viewed by friends and other family members before burial may be precluded.

As we are confronted with the legal justice system, great complexity, and often frustration, may be added to the situation. Along with the necessity for an autopsy, which may delay the funeral process, we are likely to be dealing with the police, with lawyers and with a system which, at best, tends to move more slowly than we generally desire. Having to make a deposition, having to attend an inquest or a trial, having to hear and to tell the story repeatedly, perhaps having to read about it in the newspaper, requires reliving the situation over and over again, often under stressful circumstances.

When the outcome is what one desires, then having had to endure the legal proceedings, with all their machinations and however painful and slow, perhaps may become worthwhile or at least acceptable. Indeed, it has been noted that "a family's satisfaction with the criminal justice system can substantially help them in their grief after the murder of a family member" (Shapiro, 1994, p. 267). However, if we get to the end of the road and feel that justice has not been served, then rage is likely to become outrage as we feel both betrayed and without further recourse. In such cases, the most difficult aspect of the grieving process may involve having to learn to live with a double sense of injustice, of having been victimized not once but twice.

There are other instances, however, when involvement with the legal system may provide an opportunity that enables the bereaved to feel as if they are doing something to right a wrong. This seems to be particularly true for the parents of children who have been the victims of violent or wrongful death. Thus, "In cases of wrongful deaths, parents often work tirelessly to ensure that the police and court systems bring justice to the death" (Klass, 1988, p. 38). The challenge for such parents, as well as for others, is to avoid assuming a vengeful stance and to overcome a sense of helplessness even as they continue to do everything in their power to assure an appropriate outcome. When such efforts fail, they may turn to political activism or the creation of victims' rights organizations such as Mothers Against Drunk Driving (MADD), or Parents of Murdered Children, which may provide helpful and creative ways to channel their grief. By contrast, such outlets are not so readily available in the case of suicide.

SUICIDE

Indeed, death by suicide leads to yet another situation in which the pain of the loss is confounded by a mixture of emotions experienced in response to the circumstances of the death. Whereas public awareness may be welcome and even sought in the case of violent or wrongful death, the desire for privacy may be primary when suicide is the cause of death. What is more, feelings of guilt and an inability to speak about the death because of the social stigma involved may complicate the grieving of those whose loved ones have died as a result of a completed suicide (J. R. Bernstein, 1997). Such feelings and reactions are logical given the many cultural stories about suicide which portray it as a sinful act, as representing criminal behavior, and/or as behavior that is indicative of weakness or madness (Kastenbaum, 1986). For example, "Some religions do not allow suicides to be buried on hallowed ground or religious services to be held" (Starhawk, Nightmare, & The Reclaiming Collective, 1997, p. 263).

In addition, survivors, and particularly close family members, may feel both anger at and a sense of rejection by their loved one given the lack of warning when someone they cared about succeeds in ending his or her own life (Nurmi & Williams, 1997). For parents, resentment may emerge as a result of "having been electively and publicly abandoned by a son or daughter who, in the minds of the parents, catastrophically showed that their love was not enough" (Schiff, 1977, p. 42). And even when resentment and rejection are not experienced, at the very least survivors may find themselves totally puzzled by such a choice on the part of their loved one and may spend years trying to figure out missed cues or other clues to what ultimately transpired. This is particularly true in the case of adolescent suicide:

> When someone is psychotic, has a clear terminal illness, or is spiritually and physically imprisoned, we can understand the source of this degree of present despair and complete loss of hope for the future. However, when we refer to adolescents in good physical health, with "their whole life ahead of them," it is difficult, if not impossible, to understand the thoughts underlying such a final action. (Gutstein, 1991, p. 241)

Given the likelihood of feelings of guilt, it is extremely important to help with the process of putting self-blame in perspective (Martin & Romanowski, 1994) in addition to providing support for the grief of those who are bereaved as a function of suicide. In this regard, it is important to be aware that no clear evidence exists regarding the causes of suicide. Even when notes are left, they may be ambiguous or incomplete. The act may be carefully planned or it may be spontaneous; it may be a response to either a single incident or many. Each completed suicide therefore must be understand as a unique, personal event. It also may be as much or more a statement about the person who has died as it is about those left behind. However, survivors of suicide may be in great need of professional assistance as they tend to be at higher risk for morbidity and mortality than others in the first year of bereavement (Shneidman, 1980b).

An important consideration for those working with someone who has lost a loved one as a result of a completed suicide also may involve the need to create a story about what has happened that enables things to be seen in a less negative way (Shapiro, 1994). The ability to understand the pain or confusion that the deceased person may have been experiencing, or the fact that the person may not have thought through the act in great detail, may be useful in this regard. Also helpful may be the awareness that one's final act does not negate either the entirety of that person or all the positive attributes and relationships that were created prior to his or her death.

AMBIGUOUS DEATH AND LOSS

Ambiguous death and loss occurs when there is uncertainty either about whether or not death has actually occurred or about the cause of death. Lack of public validation and prescribed rituals which aid the bereaved characterize the experience of the survivors in these situations (Boss, 1991, 1999). When family members have been absent or lost for extended periods, for example, with soldiers missing in action, or kidnapping or desertion, closure is prevented and those left behind must linger in limbo regarding the fate of their loved one. In other cases, psychological absence as a result of disease processes, drug overdose, or comas induced by accidents may create a void which produces confusion and conflict among family members.

Another type of ambiguity is illustrated when the cause of death is unable to be determined. In the initial aftermath, while police investigations are being carried on, family members may feel a need to remain circumspect in what they reveal to others. They may fear a verdict that does not mesh with their intuitive belief, for example, that it was not a suicide. When there is insufficient evidence to decide that the death has occurred by accident or as the result of a completed suicide or was caused by another person, there may be a sense of relief. However, although the family members may now go public with their thoughts and feelings, along with their grief they also must learn to accept the fact that they may never know what actually happened. All that they know is that their loved one has died.

Assisting family members in their efforts to deal with ambiguous death and loss may involve several steps (Boss, 1991, 1999). In the first place, it is important to provide empathy for and understanding of the fact that the situation is a stressful one. Second, allowing family members to express and hear each other's perceptions of the situation may be useful. Offering and clarifying as much information about the ordeal as possible is a third step in the support process. A fourth option involves putting family members in touch with support groups and others who have had similar experiences. Fifth and finally, as in all other cases of bereavement, facilitating a process of resolution through the search for and creation of meaning is essential to successfully resolving grief.

Indeed, the overriding goal seems to be that of helping family members to be resilient in the face of highly stressful circumstances. They are challenged to recreate their lives in ways that work for them in spite of the ambiguity of the situation. And although there may be lack of clarity regarding who is in and who is out of the family, or regarding how a person has died, survivors ultimately must succeed in creating a personal story that enables them to attribute meaning to the loss. All this requires support that is sensitive to the uniqueness of the situation.

PROVIDING SUPPORT FOR THE PROCESS OF RESOLUTION

Just as the importance of social support in the case of ambiguous death and loss cannot be underestimated, so also does this seem to be a common thread which runs throughout discussions of the various ways in which death, dying, and bereavement may occur and grief may be felt and resolved. However, it appears that it is the perception of support relative to its availability and degree of experienced satisfaction that is critical to its ability to ameliorate reactions to death (Reif, Patton, & Gold, 1995; Sarason, Sarason, Shearin, & Pierce, 1987). That is, although we may make efforts to help family members and other survivors who are mourning the loss of a loved one, what we do must be perceived as meaningful if it is to be helpful. Good intentions are not sufficient. Instead, we must tailor our responses to meet specific needs. It thus may be useful to consider a variety of approaches that we may take as part of the effort to provide meaningful support for those bereaved as a function of the various ways in which death may come unannounced.

Being with the Pain and Shock

One of the first gifts we may offer to those bereaved following a sudden death is a willingness coupled with an ability just to be with them and to allow them to cry, to rage, to despair, to express all their feelings. Rather than trying to soothe them or make things better, rather than getting caught up in the mundane details of daily living, we may attempt to provide a sense of real support by our presence in the midst of death and dying. Accordingly, the survivors may have an awareness that they are not alone as we allow ourselves to cry with them, to express our shock and disbelief, to talk about the person who has died, and/or to share fond memories. By so doing we may be able to contribute a sense of community as well as a sense of safety, a container for their grief, as we offer our implicit permission as well as validation for their experience, whatever it might be.

Indeed, what we must not do is to try to take away the pain or talk the bereaved out of their tears. What we must do is be ready to ride the tide of emotion when a brief moment of laughter quickly dissolves into gut-wrenching sobs. We must be willing to witness the anguish not only for this loss but also for many other losses that also may have occurred. We must be able to acknowledge with the survivors what was and can never be again. And we must accept that anger and guilt may be logical responses in the initial aftermath of an unexpected death. As they are ready over time, we may then begin to think about ways in which to help the bereaved deal appropriately with, and ultimately come to terms with, their anger.

Dealing with Anger

Anger is an essential component of grief (Shapiro, 1994) and sometimes grief is most easily and overtly expressed through anger. We may rage at the person who has died, at ourselves, at real or imagined injustice, at God, at others who may have been involved, at the lack of sensitivity of our community and larger culture. Such feelings are real, they are valid and they are important. They speak to a sense of impotence and to the difficulty we may be having in accepting the facts of a lost life and a reality gone awry.

Once again, rather than attempting to deny or to diminish the feelings, it may be useful to encourage a full exploration of the anger felt by the bereaved person. Writing, perhaps in a journal or in letters not intended to be sent, may provide a means for articulating and analyzing the depth of the emotions that have emerged. When the writing has been completed for the time being or if it is inappropriate, encouraging some kind of activity that allows for the physical expression of intense feelings (e.g., hammering) and that perhaps leads to the creation of something tangible and useful (e.g., a piece of furniture) also may prove helpful. Providing the opportunity to go into the anger and experience it fully may help to avoid the creation of the paradox in which we feel guilty about our feelings. And when the feelings are able to be fully expressed, they may in time diminish of their own accord. However, another challenge that also may have presented itself and that certainly may require attention is the issue of guilt.

Transforming Guilt

The grief process is characterized by a great deal of irrationality in terms of thoughts, feelings, and behaviors. Feelings of guilt are some of the most typical, if irrational, of the emotions experienced by the bereaved, particularly in the case of unanticipated death. As explanations are sought, so also is the search undertaken for someone to blame or to at least share responsibility for what has happened. And often we point the finger at ourselves. However irrational such feelings may be, they are part of the person's reality and need to be respected.

The first response may be to discuss the nature of the guilt and to consider whether or not it is truly deserved. It is important to remember that even if it is shown to be illogical, the feelings may persist nevertheless. In this case, we may focus on a process of transforming guilt through behavior directed at helping others. That is, one may suggest that when the guilty feelings are experienced, the bereaved person do something kind or meaningful for someone else. In this manner, the negative feeling may become a catalyst for actions following which the person is able to feel more positive about him- or herself.

In those instances in which guilt may indeed be an appropriate response, transforming it involves a different kind of process. The first step, of course, involves acknowledgment of culpability or participation in the death of another. Thereafter, we may encourage efforts to make amends, for example, through offering apologies to those most closely involved or through the provision of a service to the family or the larger community. Ultimately, however, whether the feelings that persist are illogical or logical, and indeed even if guilt is not the issue, what is probably needed most is the experience of forgiveness.

Forgiving Self and Others

Forgiveness has been called the human being's "highest need and deepest achievement" (Bushnell, cited in McCutcheon, 1995, p. 219). In other words, we have much to gain through the process of forgiveness, but finding it within ourselves to forgive also may challenge us to the depths of our being. Thus, although complete forgiveness may not always be appropriate or possible, to the degree that it is there is much to be gained through its pursuit.

For example, in the case of personal feelings of guilt, perhaps the focus may be shifted to a consideration of the things that were done right and well for and with the person who has died. Perhaps in the overall scheme of things there is a great deal about which survivors are able to feel good. Perhaps the question might be posed regarding whether the person who has died would judge the survivors as harshly as they are judging themselves. Perhaps there also can be recognition that perfection in human behavior, though often an ideal, is rarely, if ever, a reality. Indeed, we might consider that the ability to forgive oneself moves us just a shade closer to that ideal.

When the issue involves the forgiveness of others, we might do well to offer reminders that it is the one who does the forgiving who stands to gain far more than does the one forgiven. To this end, the person who is struggling with angry feelings toward someone else might be encouraged to engage in a letter-writing exercise (Deits, 1988). Accordingly, the person is invited to write a letter of forgiveness to the object of the anger as if the desire was to forgive, even though that might not be the feeling at the time. The letter is to be put in an envelope which is kept in a safe place. The writer is to read the letter out loud to him- or herself every day, making changes as appropriate, until such time as the feelings of forgiveness become real. A letter such as this may then be sent, read to the other, kept by the writer, or disposed of in some appropriate manner, depending on the circumstances.

There are, of course, situations in which forgiveness may seem virtually impossible, as in the case of violent death. However, although we certainly would not condone murder or any other form of violence, perhaps in such cases we may, at the very least, be able to offer forgiveness to others for not living up to our or society's expectations of them (Becvar, 1997). Perhaps we also might be able to recognize that although our anger is justified, it is not our place to sit in judgment of others. Indeed, in such cases we also might encourage the turning of one's attention to the pursuit of justice.

Working for Justice

The ability to participate in a process aimed at achieving justice for an act of wrongdoing may provide a useful outlet for the frustration and impotence felt when someone is killed in a violent way. Not only does it serve to divert some portion of one's attention from the pain of the loss, but it also gives one a concrete and practical focus, something to do and something to accomplish. The downside, of course, as noted earlier, is the frustration that may be experienced when the process is painfully slow and complex or when the outcome further undermines one's faith that there is such a thing as justice.

Another positive outlet for grief and anger at an injustice may be found through efforts to create a kinder, gentler, safer society, one in which others will not be victimized in the way that one's loved ones have been. Engaging in such efforts may be of little interest in the early days of the bereavement process, but over time this can become an important focus. As noted earlier, such efforts have proven particularly meaningful for the parents of children who have died violently or, for example, as the result of an accident involving drunk drivers.

If political activism has little or no appeal, there are other ways in which pursuing justice may be encouraged. Perhaps it would be meaningful for the bereaved person to offer prayers or meditations to this end. Perhaps she or he might be encouraged to volunteer on behalf of others who have been victimized in some way. Perhaps merely working to live a life of integrity, to enhance one's ability to be compassionate, may be sufficient to create a more just world and to satisfy one's desire to participate in creating such a reality. Reaching a place where this is possible, however, may require attention to the painful images of the loved one whose dying involved serious disfigurement.

Changing Painful Images

It is difficult enough to look at a loved one who has died and to realize that the person we knew is gone forever. However, when that person is not recognizable or bears on her or his body the effects of fatal injuries, the impact may be traumatic indeed. We may be haunted thereafter by this final mental picture which also conjures up anguish about the circumstances of the person's dying. It thus may be important to encourage efforts to replace the painful image with one that is more consistent with the person she or he was when vital and healthy.

One relatively simple tactic may be to keep lots of photographs out and around the house. Or we may create a photograph album and keep it handy so that we can remind ourselves of the way the loved one really looked when alive. As the painful image comes into awareness, we can turn to a picture and have a tangible reminder. We might also smile at the picture and say, out loud or to ourselves, words of endearment or affection, such as "I love you," or "I miss you." We might also imagine the person in the picture smiling back.

Another approach may be found in the use of guided imagery, directed either by the self or by another. In this case, the person brings to mind the final painful image. Guidance is then given, slowly, to engage in a process of changing each feature, each disfigurement, until the person is once more seen as whole. This is to be a gentle, loving, healing process, which enables the survivor to feel as though she or he is actually ministering to the one who has died. Although there is no denial that death has occurred, ideally more acceptable images of both self and other are thereby created. Although perhaps the most elusive, the need to change painful images may be one of the most important pieces of unfinished business requiring attention. However, there certainly may be other loose ends that also need tying up.

Tying Up Loose Ends

Given the suddenness of the death, survivors may experience a sense that many issues just have been left hanging in midair. This may be particularly true for unfinished business in the realm of relationships. Perhaps there were harsh words spoken in the final days, or unfulfilled promises. Perhaps there were old animosities about which the survivor has regrets. Perhaps there are a variety of thoughts and feelings we wish there had been time or opportunity to express. Whether the loose ends are trivial or momentous, they nevertheless deserve time and attention in order to achieve a sense of completion.

Once again, letter writing may prove to be helpful. However, in this case the letter written is to the one who has died. In the letter, the bereaved person shares his or her thoughts, feelings, wishes, or whatever seems most appropriate. This is to be a careful and thoughtful process. When the letter is completed, the bereaved may wish to read it out loud to the person who has died. The reading of the letter may be done at home, in a special place that was meaningful. Or, the person may wish to go to the cemetery and read it there if this would seem to foster a greater sense of connection and a feeling that the message is being received.

A person for whom letter writing does not seem suitable may be invited to just speak his or her thoughts to the one who has died, either silently or out loud. This also may be done at the graveside. Another option may be to find a peaceful place where there will be no disturbances for a time. Holding something that belonged to the loved one, the bereaved person may be encouraged to go into a receptive or meditative state. The person may then "share" his or her thoughts with the one who has died. Although there may be no confirmation from the recipient, the process may foster a sense of peace about the effort to tie up loose ends. Indeed, this may be one important aspect of creating positive stories, whether about oneself, about the one who has died, or about death in general.

Creating Positive Stories

If the characteristic that is most unique in the case of sudden and accidental death is the assault to our belief system, then the challenge most in
need of attention at some point in the grieving process is that of recreating our worldview. And certainly we will be served best by stories that enable us to see whatever has happened in the most positive light possible.
However, such a need is likely to be present to some degree whenever we
find ourselves in the presence of grief. Therefore, Chapter 12 is devoted to
discussions of ways in which we may help the bereaved make meaning out
of what initially may be experienced as meaningless, senseless events. In
the meantime, the next chapter considers deaths which are anticipated.

THERAPEUTIC CONVERSATIONS
AND REFLECTIONS

Louise and Harry, a 30-something couple, took their three young
children for a weekend at a nearby beach where they all enjoyed
boating and fishing. Both parents were heavily involved in careers
which required a lot of travel, so family time such as this was important and they planned outings whenever possible. By midafternoon
on Sunday the children had had enough fishing and swimming and
were content to play at the edge of the water. Harry decided to go
for one last fishing venture before it was time to return home.

Louise stayed with the children, periodically looking up to
watch her husband. After about a half hour, she realized could no
longer see Harry although his boat was still visible. At first she
thought that he must have jumped into the water for a swim or was
leaning over to fix something. As time passed, however, and still she
saw no sign of him, she became concerned. The distance was too
great to be able to call to her husband so she looked around for
someone who might be able to help.

Louise explained the situation to two men in a nearby boat,
asking them to go out to her husband and investigate. With a sink-
ing heart and growing fear, she watched as the men reached her husband's boat, bending over as they climbed into it. After some time,
the two men began towing Harry's boat back to shore. By this time,

(cont.)

---

a curious crowd was gathering. Fearful about her husband and worried about alarming the children, she asked an acquaintance to take the children for ice cream. When the boats arrived, Harry was lifted out and laid on the shore. Someone performed CPR and an ambulance was called, but to no avail. Harry apparently had died instantly, although the cause would have to be determined.

As Louise told me this story, several months later, she was in a state of shock and despair. She couldn't remember how she had managed to get through the first days and weeks, although she knew that people had been very kind and had helped enormously in terms of caring for the children and notifying family members and friends. Her mother had come to stay with the family for 3 weeks but she had had to go home in order to care for her husband, Louise's stepfather, who was seriously ill. Since then, Louise had gone back to work but found that her job had lost much of its previous excitement and allure. She worried about the children and the need to be able to spend more time with them. Although the family's financial situation enabled Louise to consider taking a leave or even quitting her job, she feared being at home fulltime would be more than she could bear. Most significant, however, in addition to her great sadness, was Louise's anger—both at her husband and at herself.

Harry had died of heart failure. As both had known, Harry's family had a long history of heart disease and, in fact, Harry's father had died when he was just a few years younger than Harry had been at the time of his death. Louise had often asked Harry to pay closer attention to his diet, to get more frequent checkups, to exercise more. However, she had not pushed as hard as she might have and he had not really paid too much attention to her. He had been so focused on career and family and had felt so fit that he really didn't think his health was an issue.

Initially it seemed important just to let Louise express her anger, her sadness, her feelings of guilt, her confusion. We also spent time discussing the children, beginning the process of sorting out her concerns about their well-being. Eventually, Louise decided that she would take a 6-month leave from work in order to be able to have more time at home, give herself an opportunity to heal before making any major career decisions, and provide space to focus on her grief and the assorted emotions she was experiencing. During this period I requested that Louise keep a journal of her thoughts and feelings.

Overcoming guilt and resolving her anger were major stumbling blocks for Louise. However, an important turning point occurred when she was able to recognize, through her writing, that her husband had died as he had lived—full of life, optimistic, happy, at peace with the world. It was this ability to trust and to feel secure that she had most loved about him. What is more, he had been a good husband, a good father, and a good provider for the family. Rather than continuing to beat herself up and rage at him for what he didn't do, she began to appreciate once again who he was and what he did do. She also acknowledged that her reticence in speaking about health concerns had been her way of respecting his choices. Once Louise had reached this point, I encouraged her to write a letter to her husband, letting him know of her struggles and pain, her gratitude for what they had shared, and forgiving both of them for not having made different choices.

I am fully aware that forgiveness did not erase the pain for this young woman, nor was it easily achieved. However, once it became possible, it seemed to ease a great burden that was complicating her grief. And as Louise created a story about Harry and their relationship that acknowledged its strengths and gifts, she was able to feel sad, to miss him, and at the same to begin the process of re-creating her life. In time, she decided that a full-time career was in everyone's best interests and she resumed her work. Today she continues the search for answers and is slowly gaining a greater perspective that enables her to take care of herself and her children while learning to live fully once again. We now meet on a monthly basis, an arrangement that Louise feels is very supportive.

CHAPTER 4

When Death Is Anticipated

∽

My brother died of colon cancer in December 1965. His death was preceded by 9 months of treatment in two phases. In the first phase he had surgery for removal of a portion of his colon and the construction of a colostomy. After this initial treatment, he returned home for 3 months. At that time, we all anticipated a full recovery.

As it turned out, however, this hope was short-lived because in September he experienced more problems. He entered the hospital for the complete removal of his colon and an ileostomy. Complications of this treatment and circulatory problems led to the amputation of his left leg below the knee.

The contrasts between the two phases of my brother's illness were great. In the first phase, I made several visits. Our discussions together were upbeat and included thoughts about his plans to return to work and to resume his normal life with his family. While these conversations were enjoyable, they were not unusual in my relationship with him. He was 15 years my senior, and although I respected him as my older brother, the designation of sibling seemed much more appropriate than did the designation brother.

It was during the second phase of his illness that we truly became brothers. His wife and daughter lived a greater distance from the hospital where he was being treated than I did. Also, his wife was required to work to keep the family going. I was the one who was able to go to the hospital more regularly and was privileged to enjoy many long periods alone with him as I visited each weekend from September until November, when he returned home. Our interactions during this period were rich, deep, and personal and we came to really know each other for the first time. Life and death were topics of conversation as were his concerns for the well-being of his wife and daughter. These times of intimate sharing were spiritual experiences for both of us.

Yes, our conversations represented a spiritual experience and they were wonderful. However, the whole process was also extremely painful. I was getting to know my brother for the first time in my life, and the dark cloud of his illness threatened to take this newfound relationship away from me. I wanted to hang on to it, and yet I knew that it could be snatched away from me at any time. And it was.

In October, my brother was given approximately 6 more months to live. I recall my first reaction as deep sadness. At the same time, there also was a feeling in me of denial. Six months seemed like a long time, and, I believed naively, a time for hope that he might yet recover. What I found most interesting was his positive attitude with visitors other than myself. With me, on the other hand, he seemed to be able to feel the full depth and variety of his emotions. I felt privileged to be able to experience this courageous man.

When he returned home in November, my visits became less frequent and our conversations were somewhat different from what they had been in the hospital. I wanted more. I wanted more of my brother and his rich experience and wisdom. But he did what he had to do. He focused on putting his worldly affairs in order and making his peace with his God and his family.

When he died in December, the flurry of activity around my brother's funeral and the gathering of family and friends masked the void that I felt without his physical presence. I did what I could to help his wife and daughter as he had asked me to do. Life went on as it does. But while time may help, it does not fill voids. I feel his presence every day and yet I miss his companionship, which so enriched my life for the four short months before he died.

It has been 24 years since my brother's death. Although he is no longer in this reality, he is still very much a part of my world. It is a rare day when I do not think about him and feel blessed for having had the opportunity to get to know him. If he had died suddenly, without the time anticipating his death, I know I would have missed him, but I would not have been missing the man I came to know. In those final months, I had the privilege of witnessing a measure of courage in dealing with pain and loss of hope of recovery that I had not seen before. For example, I recall the celebration of his birthday in the middle of the second phase of his illness. Even as he neared the end of his life he was able to be upbeat and entertaining for the benefit of his daughter, who at the time was only 13.

Today my brother continues to enrich my life, particularly in moments of discouragement, when I experience again his courage, perseverance, and concern for others. It is also in these moments that I feel his presence most strongly.

—R J B

When death is anticipated or follows an extended illness, a different variety of issues rises to the fore. In this case, the grieving process may involve not only the survivors but also the one who is dying. Above all, at the point of a terminal diagnosis the person who is ill confronts and ultimately must reconcile him- or herself to, the fact of his or her own imminent demise. Given this awareness she or he also is faced with the challenge of dealing with and attempting to put in order various details related to areas such as family, finances, and life aspirations. And the dying person is forced to think about the circumstances of his or her death, which certainly may be frightening, or at least overwhelming, to contemplate.

Not surprisingly, the knowledge that the end is near generally initiates a period of anticipatory mourning not only for the dying person but also for family and friends. In the context of the inescapable fact that a loss is at hand, as noted previously, the experience of bereavement may begin even though the person is still very much alive (Rolland, 1991) and despite the fact that the dying person may or may not want to focus on death. What is more, those who take on the role of caretaker for the person who is ill are likely to experience the stress involved with both varied emotional responses and major physical responsibilities. It also is not unusual in such circumstances of increased stress for problematic family patterns to be heightened. And such family dynamics may be particularly challenging if the illness of the person who is dying carries with it a social stigma as, for example, in the case of AIDS. Also added to the mix is the fact that regardless of the type of illness, the person who is dying may worry about becoming a burden because of such things as the care required, the cost of treatments involved, and the reduced ability to be a source of income.

Finally, when the anticipated death ultimately occurs, it may bring with it a whole new set of feelings and reactions. On the one hand, there may be sadness and grief, and perhaps confusion, that there is so much pain when everyone theoretically was prepared for the loss. On the other hand, there may be relief that death finally has come and the ordeal has ended. Taken together, these conflicting emotions may produce guilt and remorse, despite the fact that they are normal and quite predictable responses.

Despite such challenges, however, there also are some benefits to be derived from having an awareness that the time of death is near. The person who is ill has a chance to give attention to any unfinished business in his or her life. What is more, the person may have input into and even may design his or her own dying process. For example, the person may participate in decisions about how much medical intervention there is to be, who is to make health-related decisions when and if she is unable, as well as how her body is to be handled after death. The person may express preferences regarding the type of funeral desired and may specify the details if so inclined. There is also a potential for achieving closure and perhaps reconciliation in significant relationships. Indeed, the dying person may be able to express his or her final wishes in all aspects of his or her life. Moreover, the dying person is afforded an opportunity to reflect on the life just lived, to assess accomplishments, and even to achieve some final goals or dreams. Everyone else involved also is given time to assimilate what is happening and to begin the process of realigning beliefs and meaning systems as they seek to come to terms with the death of a loved one.

Many of the characteristics of an anticipated death to which we just briefly have alluded remain the same regardless of life stage, but clearly distinct needs and concerns emerge when the dying person is a child. For example, consideration must be given to what the child is able to understand, which therefore influences the degree and kind of information to be shared with the child. Such consideration also must include the child's siblings and the impact on them of having and/or watching a sister or brother die. When the person who is terminally ill is a child there are likely to be few ends that need to be tied up, as is often the situation with dying persons who have reached adulthood. Nevertheless, there still may be relationship issues to be resolved or relieved as well as a need for sensitivity to patterns of behavior among family members that are likely to be stimulated by the crisis of the terminal illness and impending death.

In all cases of anticipated death, however, the goal is to create a context that enables the dying person to live as fully as possible while facilitating her or his ability to die well. It also includes awareness of and attention to the needs of caregivers and other family members who are being affected by the illness and the loss. Thus, for example, it may be important to be able to learn to savor and make the most of moments of enjoyment whenever and wherever they occur. In addition, encouraging a willingness to be present to the dying process may provide an experience of healing that enables all participants to bear their grief more easily. And taking advantage of the opportunity afforded to speak one's farewells may add grace and beauty to what previously might have been considered or expected to be an unlovely experience.

In this chapter we therefore focus on four main areas. The first focus is that of the period of the extended illness and the impact of having knowledge about an impending death on the one who is ill as well as on caregivers and other family members and friends. The second focus is the process of preparation that the dying person may be encouraged to engage in as she or he nears the end of life. The third focus is that of variations that may occur and require attention when the goal is that of supporting children who are dying. And, finally, this chapter concludes with a focus on living fully and dying well, which includes not only the one who is dying but also the other participants in this process. Throughout the discussions in each of these areas, this chapter addresses the ramifications of various behaviors for the grief process that follows the death that is anticipated.

THE EXTENDED ILLNESS

To be given the news, or confirmation of fears, that one is dying generally is to receive the ultimate blow to one's personhood or sense of self. In a single instant that individual is faced with the stark reality of his own mortality, an awareness that he may have worked hard to avoid altogether, or at least keep at bay. The person confronts the unavoidable fact that soon he will no longer be, at least as he has known himself in this lifetime. Never again will the person be able to anticipate and strive for sought-after goals and dreams. What is more, he knows that soon he will be leaving behind all he holds dear. He will not be there for future important events in the lives of those whom he loves. And he also will not be there to provide support for loved ones if and when they are in need.

It is at this point that the dying person, as well as the members of his or her support system, may begin moving through Kübler-Ross's (1969) five stages: denial, rage and anger, bargaining, depression and acceptance. Indeed, news of our own end is nearly inconceivable to comprehend, at least at first or unless one has "practiced dying," for example, as part of a spiritual discipline (Levine, 1997). And even in the latter instance, though certainly we may attempt to prepare ourselves, we cannot really know how we will feel until the moment when we actually experience it, when we truly come face to face with the fact of our dying. Denial is thus a logical response to news that is difficult or seemingly impossible to assimilate. Indeed, words such as the following, spoken in response to a terminal cancer diagnosis and the reactions of several physicians that no treatments are available, are therefore rather typical: "I won't take no for an answer. It's bullshit. I'm fifty-four. I'm not ready to just pack it up and die. I'm a fighter. I don't buy that *nothing* can be done" (Groopman, 1997, p. 7).

Family members and friends may be challenged in a similar manner as they struggle with their own shock and disbelief. Their denial may arise out of both an inability to accept the knowledge that a loved one is dying and fears for their own well-being that may be triggered by this information. On the one hand, there is the pain of knowing the other person is about to die, that the relationship with that person will soon be over, that one will be left behind, and so on. On the other hand, accepting the fact that a loved one is dying brings home in a personal way the awareness of our own mortality.

When the day comes that the inevitable is acknowledged, anger at any one of a number of things—the situation, God, perceived injustice, the self, and/or others for supposed failures or shortcomings—often replaces the denial. In addition, all the stresses of the situation are likely to lead to more volatile tempers and shorter fuses, thereby intensifying the context of anger. Therefore, a range of moods is highly likely as the individuals involved alternately grieve for what cannot be and rage against what they do not want.

As the anger begins to subside, the bargaining phase may be initiated. That is, the dying person may believe, or perhaps hope, that if she has somehow fallen short given her own or another's assessment of herself, then doing something more or better may change the course of events in a favorable manner. A commitment to offer a service or somehow provide for others, or perhaps in some way to make amends for a past wrong may therefore be offered in return for the promise, or at least the potential, of a cure at best and a longer life at worst. Other members of the dying person's support network also may participate in similar kinds of bargaining processes.

It is important to note here that both of these stages of emotional response—denial and bargaining—not only are normal but also may be important catalysts to healing. According to research into some forms of cancer (Siegel, 1986), those who do best in terms of long-term survival are the fighters. Those who do the next best are the patients who deny. For example, in the instance of the man who was given the terminal cancer diagnosis whose words of disbelief were quoted earlier, aggressive therapy was undertaken and, much to everyone's surprise, he achieved a complete remission. Although the cancer ultimately returned, at which point it proved fatal, the man had been able to return to a full normal life for another year following his initial treatment (Groopman, 1997).

Indeed, as Cousins (1989) notes, there is no way of knowing that hope might not be helpful and appropriate. None of us can ever really be certain of the outcome until it has occurred. And even if this outcome turns out to be death, the willingness to fight for one's life may prove to have been an important aspect of the healing process through recognition and a sense of satisfaction about the fact that one has done everything possible to maintain life in the best way one knows how.

Nevertheless, when all avenues have been explored, all options exhausted, and the inexorable movement toward the final days of life has begun, there comes a point when acceptance is not only appropriate but also likely to be beneficial. Now one can truly focus on the awareness of death and make every effort to do whatever is necessary to be at peace when the last breath is breathed. As discussed in succeeding sections, acceptance in this case is an active rather than a passive process. Before giving further consideration to this final phase of the dying process, however, it is important to be aware of the continuing impact on caregivers and other friends and family members as each of these phases is negotiated.

Some of the most important decisions that must be made concern where the person who is ill will die (e.g., at home or in the hospital) and how others will be involved. If the person desires to die at home, arrangements must be made for appropriate medical supervision and caregivers must be designated. Also of concern are the daily lives of immediate family members who are most affected. For example, if one parent is the primary caregiver for the other parent who is the person dying, attention must be given to the needs of children and the general running of the household. Or, if the dying person is in the hospital, the need to be present both there and at home may tax the endurance of even the most hardy. In the case of an elderly couple, the requirements of care simply may be more than can be handled alone by the spouse who is not dying. In other words, regardless of the situation, the strain on caregivers is enormous and must be acknowledged and dealt with effectively. Everyone also must be aware that the context within which they are operating is one of sadness and grief at the impending loss.

How the multitude of important issues are addressed and the various challenges are faced by family members and friends will be greatly influenced by already well-established relationship patterns. If mutual support and generosity are the norm, the stresses and strains are likely to be managed in an optimal manner. People will respond when called on and also may pitch in without being asked. Even when conflict arises, as it inevitably will, it will be dealt with effectively and then everyone will move on without lasting damage to relationships. Generally speaking, decisions will be negotiated respectfully and the experience will be a basically satisfying one despite the circumstances.

If there are underlying tensions and old hostilities, however, they certainly will emerge around the crisis of the anticipated death. Unfortunately, such patterns are likely not only to impede the process but also to be exacerbated by the demands of the situation. What is more, such negative patterns will tend both to detract from the experience of the person who is dying and to divert the focus from that which is most essential in the final days of that person's life and beyond. In other words, rather than concentration on the grief over the loss, the primary emotion tends to be anger at family members, which does little to honor the person who is dying or has died.

Indeed, families may be torn apart as a function of unresolved conflicts which surface in the context of the death of a loved one. And this certainly can occur with any kind of terminal condition or circumstances of dying. For example, it may involve disagreements over care during the dying person's final days. It may involve failure to notify family members that the final moments of life are at hand. It may involve exclusion of one or more family members in the making of important decisions related to participation in final rituals, for example which of several children is to be given the opportunity, or not, to speak at their father's funeral. It may involve fierce fighting over furniture or other possessions owned by the deceased. Perhaps the most severe forms of conflict, however, are evident in situations in which an illness carries with it a social stigma and/or taps into deeply held beliefs and feelings.

For example, in the case of AIDS, spouses may be split by their differing responses as one parent chooses to care for a dying son and the other parent chooses to remain separate, perhaps not even visit, because of negative feelings about that son's homosexuality. Conversely, the parents may stand staunchly by their child but may be shunned by extended family members and former friends, who refuse to attend the funeral or acknowledge the death in any way. Indeed, some parents may feel compelled to hide the cause of death because of their fear of rejection by friends and family members (Nolen-Hoeksema & Larson, 1999).

Regardless of the particular scenario and the degree of hostility or emotional and physical distancing, lack of support and an absence of mutual respect and solidarity through the crisis both detract from the dying process and add to the grief experience (Shapiro, 1994). Thus, to whatever extent possible, it is crucial to pay attention to all dimensions—body, mind, spirit—from the moment of diagnosis and continuing long after the death has occurred. And despite the various challenges, it is important to be aware that much can be done to enable the person who is ill to make the most of her or his final days and to facilitate, for all the participants, healing in the midst of dying. Thus, I next consider some of the important aspects of preparation for dying.

THE PROCESS OF PREPARATION

In his book *Who Dies?*, poet and meditation teacher Stephen Levine (1982, p. 5) asks: "Who is prepared to die? Who has lived so fully that they are not threatened by their imaginings of nonexistence?" What we fear most, according to Levine, is the idea of death and our sense of a loss of control over what happens after death. However, it is also his belief that what we have is a choice. We can allow our fear of the unknown to constrict us to the point that we are unable to do little more than die, with much left unsaid and unresolved. Or, we can open up to and explore that which is unknown and allow our dying to be a door to a sense of peace and serenity as we enter into the great mystery with an open heart and an accepting spirit.

Clearly, although always a daunting undertaking, making the latter choice is more difficult to do if we have not given much thought to our dying before receiving a terminal diagnosis. However, even if we come with little prior attention to the awareness that life is about to end, the anticipated death affords us some precious time to make ourselves ready if we are willing. At the same time, in either case there most probably will be moments of doubt and fear, times when one's faith is sorely tested. Indeed, it is in the realm of faith and belief that we may meet our most difficult challenges.

That is, although it is the physical body that often is the major focus of attention, the part of us that ultimately gives out, it is at the spiritual level that our beingness truly is called into question. And it is through the mind that we build a bridge that enables us to make of the final journey either a unique and special experience to be celebrated or just one more mundane event simply to be endured. Clearly, then, an equally important focus is the belief system of the dying person.

Gentle explorations of thoughts about what happens after we die and the provision of opportunities to discuss fears and consider new ideas thus may be helpful for the one who is terminally ill. It also may be appropriate to suggest books to be read, either by the dying person him- or herself or aloud by caregivers. Seeking information or support from a clergy person or spiritual guide might be considered as well. But regardless of the way chosen, which is explored in more depth in the final section of this chapter, what is important is awareness of the spiritual dimension of the dying process. Also crucial is a willingness to support and facilitate whatever would be most helpful for the person as he or she mentally prepares for death.

Not surprisingly, however, a focus on things spiritual often is postponed until closure has been achieved with regard to some of the more practical issues. Generally we tend to think, at least initially, that putting our affairs in order requires most of all a consideration of financial and legal issues. Certainly these, too, are important, and also are often in need of attention. That is, in the ongoing effort to avoid the inevitable, many come to their final days without having made a will or designated someone who is to have power of attorney or be the executor of their estate. And even when such legalities have been attended to, there may have been little sharing about where important documents are kept, for example, or little awareness on the part of close family members regarding their financial status. It therefore behooves the dying person and her or his immediate family to sort out what needs to be done, to see that affairs are put in order, and to keep everyone as fully informed as possible and appropriate.

Recent years have seen a growing awareness of the need to make plans and formally express one's wishes regarding the extent and kind of treatment desired, particularly during the last phase of dying. One may therefore wish to complete a living will and/or may designate a health care proxy by creating a durable power of attorney for health care. In the latter case, the goal is to appoint a specific person who will make sure that the medical decisions made are consistent with what the dying person would choose if she or he were capable of doing so for her- or himself. The dying person is thus able to specify when and if life-sustaining treatment is to be withdrawn as well as make a request that medication and other measures be limited to maintaining comfort and relieving pain. In addition, the person may describe the specific forms of treatment that will or will not be acceptable (e.g., cardiac resuscitation, mechanical respiration, tube feeding, blood transfusions, surgery, invasive diagnostic tests, kidney dialysis, and/or antibiotics).

Depending on the type of illness and the degree to which various areas of the body are likely to be affected, one also may wish to consider organ donation. In some cases, the choice even may be to donate one's entire body for purposes of scientific research. These are delicate areas, however, and need to be broached with care, especially if the discussion is not initiated by the person who is ill. At the same time, that person may feel strongly about preferences in this regard and may be grateful to have such issues brought to his or her attention. For, with everything that comes flooding in, it certainly is possible that important details such as these may be inadvertently or unintentionally overlooked.

Some of the other concerns that may be uppermost in the mind of the dying person fall into a far less tangible realm. These include the sense of accomplishment one may feel, or the lack thereof, as the life just lived is reviewed and assessed. Brought home most intensely at this time may be the developmental issues of the stage of maturity described as ego integrity versus despair by (Erikson, 1963). That is, has the person accomplished what she or he set out to do? Have the goals she or he deemed most important been achieved? If so, the person may experience a sense of accomplishment and completion that enables both satisfaction with life and acceptance of death. Or, is there a feeling that one's life was lived in a rather superficial manner, that few contributions of real value were made in any area? Is there an awareness that much precious time was wasted, that given another chance one would live life in a very different way? If the person is still quite young, is there a sense of having been cheated of life's opportunities? In situations such as these, the person may sink into depression and despair, dying emotionally long before physical death occurs.

Awareness of the likelihood of such reflections and their potential impact may alert caregivers to the need for attention, perhaps from professionals, to the mental and emotional realm. Such attention may enable the dying person to come to terms with her or his life in a way that avoids discouragement and provides the potential for a more positive assessment. Having someone with whom to discuss feelings about hopes and dreams, particularly those which have not been fulfilled, may allow for the creation of a broader or different perspective, one that permits the dying person to acknowledge areas in which success was achieved. In addition, through conversation and reflection on what has been missing, the dying person may recognize that there is still time to meet some personal desires, either for her- or himself or for loved ones.

It is much more likely that dying persons will be able to express, without much prompting, thoughts about the type of funeral desired. They may have detailed requests regarding the location of the service, the selection of music, the choice between burial and cremation. If burial is preferred, consideration also must be given to whether or not the casket is to be open or closed. If cremation is the choice, there may be a strong preference regarding the disposal of the ashes. Some may want their ashes buried in a cemetery or a columbarium, whereas others may wish their ashes to be scattered in a favorite or otherwise significant place.

At the same time, there are certainly many instances in which the person who is dying may neither initiate nor wish to discuss any of these kinds of issues. And whether such discussion is possible or not, family members face a considerable challenge either as they attempt to talk when conversation is desired or possible or as they are faced with having to make decisions for the person who is terminally ill in the context of their own pain and grief. However, once again, the opportunity also exists to make this challenge a means of bringing closure to relationships in such a way that everyone benefits.

For those who are about to lose someone to death, knowing in advance allows space to work toward the healing of old wounds by expressing or asking for forgiveness. Or the moment might now seem right to share important information that was long withheld for a variety of reasons. Time for discussion and mutual consideration of issues in an open and honest way may pave the way for the creation of compromise and goodwill where previously there was emotional distancing and/or open hostility. Knowing that this may be the last opportunity to speak, to resolve differences, may enable everyone to venture into areas previously avoided or at least tiptoed around.

The dying person also may seek to take advantage of the final phase of life by initiating efforts at reconciliation with various important people in his or her life. The importance of being sensitive to needs in this area cannot be overemphasized. Indeed, according to some, "Dying people develop an awareness that they need to be at peace. As death nears, people often realize some things feel unfinished or incomplete—perhaps issues that once seemed insignificant or that happened long ago. Now the dying person realizes their importance and wants to settle them" (Callanan & Kelley, 1992, p. 140).

What is more, this need to be at peace, to achieve some level of reconciliation in relationships, may even be so great that death remains elusive until the goal has been attained (Callanan & Kelley, 1992)—hence the not uncommon experience in which the dying person lingers close to death for a long time. Although nothing else seems to change, when the death finally occurs it does so after an important encounter, one for which the dying person seems to have been waiting. Ideally, such closure is able to be achieved when one is in the earlier stages of dying and can be more present to and enjoy more fully the benefits of the process. But even when this is not what happens—even when the dying person is unconscious—there seems to be some level of awareness that resolution has been achieved.

Finally, also provided by the foreknowledge of death are time and the opportunity for final messages and expressions of gratitude. The dying person may wish to thank those in his or her life for various gifts, both literal and figurative, of which he or she has been a recipient. And those who will be left behind also may seize the moment in order to share their thoughts, either verbally or in writing, about what it is they most appreciated in the person who is dying. They also may wish to offer their support as the end draws near.

To illustrate, a young woman traveled across the country to be the donor for her sister who was about to undergo a bone marrow transplant. Although the transplant was deemed to have been successful, the sister contracted pneumonia shortly thereafter and it soon became apparent that she was dying. Although they were far from home, the young woman had enough time to invite family members and friends to send cards or telephone her at the hospital with whatever messages of gratitude and wishes for serenity and peace they desired to convey. Thus, in the final hours of her sister's life, the young woman was able to read and relay expressions of love and caring sent from all over the country, from young children to middle-age friends to aging family members. This was an experience that enabled the dying to take place in a context of dignity and grace that was both helpful and healing for all. Certainly this is a goal whose achievement is worthy of pursuit, both when the dying person is an adult and when the life that is ending is that of a child.

SUPPORTING DYING CHILDREN

According to Kübler-Ross (1995), "There is no one dying, whether he is five or ninety-five, who does not know that he is dying. And the question is not: do I tell him that he is dying? The question is: Can I hear him?" (p. 7). The fact is, however, that broaching the subject of death may be particularly difficult for the parents of terminally ill children. In the first place, they themselves may be in denial and thus may be unable to accept the fact that their child is dying. They also may not want to give up the last shreds of hope, and they certainly don't wish to cloud in any way the final days of their child's life. Nevertheless, sometimes it is the silence, the inability for the child to speak or the unwillingness of the parents to hear, that may be more difficult for the child than is the knowledge of her or his illness and impending death.

In contrast to most adults, terminally ill children are not as likely to have loose ends in need of tying up in a variety of areas. Further, thoughts and beliefs about death and dying may not be nearly as anxiety provoking as they are for their parents of for others who have lived longer. Thus, for them preparation for dying may require primarily a context in which they are able to express their frustrations and anger about being ill, speak their fears about dying, convey various messages to family members, and perhaps have the opportunity to fulfill a long-held goal or dream. As work with this population seems to have revealed, "Unlike older patients, the children had not accumulated layers of 'unfinished business.' They did not have a lifetime of botched relationships or a resume of mistakes. Nor did they feel compelled to pretend that everything was okay. They knew instinctively how sick they were, or that they actually were dying, and they did not hide their feelings about it" (Kübler-Ross, 1997, p. 182).

As parents attempt to figure out how to be with and how to respond to their dying child, however, they also must take into consideration other children in the family and the effect that various decisions are likely to have on them. For example, they must decide how much information is to be shared and with whom. Being direct and honest may seem the wisest course in many instances, but the ability of young children to understand what is happening must be considered. Further, when discussing the illness and issues related to death and dying, parents and caregivers must attempt to be matter of fact and to avoid engendering fear. At the same time, it is important to be aware that when the option to share the truth is chosen, siblings may be given the opportunity not only to understand what is going on but also to say their good-byes to their brother or sister. What is more, they may succeed in becoming comfortable with the idea of death, perhaps more easily than their parents.

When questions about death and dying arise, as they most definitely will, parents also must have or come up with satisfactory answers in an area in which they themselves may have little certainty. And they are challenged to find understandable ways to describe a complex topic. As is usually the best policy with children, replies that are honest, short, and simple generally will satisfy the curiosity of the moment. Also important to remember is the wisdom of acknowledging when one doesn't have answers rather than creating stories in which the parents really don't believe.

Parents also must weigh the relative merits of trying to care for their child in the home as opposed to the hospital. Issues to be taken into consideration include the resources available to support either of these choices as well as their potential impact on others in the family. For example, if one or both parents must be away from the home for extended periods, it must be possible to arrange for the care of other children. Or, conversely, if the terminally ill child is allowed to remain at home, her or his dying must be able to be managed in such a way that neither the presence of other children detracts from it nor are these other children negatively affected by it.

Indeed, a major task for parents is that of balancing the needs of the dying child with those of their other children. Regardless of their ability to understand what is going on, siblings also require time and attention both to satisfy their basic normal needs and to enable them to successfully handle their feelings of sadness, confusion or grief. Always sensitive to what is happening around them, they also may be acutely aware of what their parents may be experiencing emotionally.

This brings us, finally, to a recognition of the necessity for parents also to find ways to care for themselves. Being a parent is demanding under the best of circumstances. Being the parent of a dying child is likely to push a parent almost beyond endurance. Thus, having the opportunity to speak about their feelings and fears, being provided with respite care so they may take a break, grabbing moments whenever they are available to do something kind for themselves are all essential to the ability of parents to successfully navigate the troubled waters of their lives.

It is therefore easy to see that the need for external support from relatives, friends, and professionals may never be greater than when a family with children is dealing with the terminal illness of one of its younger members. And certainly it is not unusual for children who are ill to be tuned into and aware of the pressures and strains other family members, and particularly their parents, are experiencing and for these children to attempt to protect family members by not sharing their feelings or their level of awareness (e.g., in some situations children seem to wait to die until their parents are not in the room in order to spare them any further distress).

At the same time, and depending on their age, some children may choose to be vocal about their needs and desires. They may wish to have a say in whether or not toxic treatments are to be continued and where their dying is to take place. In addition, as they move into adolescence they may wish to be consulted regarding funeral and burial arrangements just as adults are. And they, too, may have some unresolved relationship issues. For example, in the case of a divorce, there may have been es-trangement between the noncustodial parent and other children. As the child approaches death, she or he may feel a need to have some contact with that parent, even if no words are spoken (Callanan & Kelley, 1992)

Dying children also may have a final wish that parents may seek to have fulfilled. In addition to various foundations available in this regard, particularly when the requests are beyond the means of the family to ful-fill, friends and extended family members also may be called on to make smaller dreams come true. Thus, arrangements might be made for a child to have a ride on a fire engine, visit an amusement park, or just to be able to ride his or her bike. What is important here is the ability to acknowl-edge that the end is near and hear what it is that would bring meaning to the final days of the child's life. Indeed, this applies to adults as well as children as we seek to enable the dying person, whatever his or her age, to live fully and die well.

LIVING FULLY AND DYING WELL

According to Ira Byock (1997), a staunch supporter of the hospice move-ment in this country, dying may be understood as a developmental process similar to the one that is initiated at birth. This developmental process is one the family may both support and be influenced by as the dying person moves through each stage of growth and gains a sense of mastery and ac-complishment as he or she achieves goals. Byock (1997) writes:

> People who are dying often feel a sense of constant pressure to adapt to un-wanted change. As a person's functioning declines, the physical environ-ment becomes threatening. A trip to the bathroom may become an hour's chore and then, a few weeks later, a major event. On learning of the grave prognosis, family and friends may begin acting differently, becoming serious or even solemn in one's presence. People may avoid one out of their own emotional pain, leaving one feeling awkward and isolated, an innocent pa-riah. New strategies are urgently needed to forestall a sense of personal anni-hilation. Mastering the taskwork may involve personal struggle, and even

suffering, yet it can lead to growth and dying well. The tasks are not easy. But as a dying persons reaches developmental landmarks such as experienced love of self and others, the completion of relationships, the acceptance of the finality of one's life, and the achievement of a new sense of self despite one's impending demise, one's life and the lives of others are enriched. (p. 33)

Facilitating a good death, one that enables growth and development throughout the dying process and beyond, requires attention in all the areas previously discussed. However, what seems to be most significant is a consciousness about the experience, a recognition of the sacredness of the event, a sacredness that does not necessarily refer to a religious dimension. The goal is acceptance and support of this final rite of passage by allowing what is happening, both as one dies and as others participate, to be uppermost in the awareness of everyone involved. Indeed, whether what is sought is the ultimate spiritual transformation described by deathing (Foos-Graber, 1989) or the creation of a context that simply provides peace and serenity, death and dying become a ceremony in which one is privileged to share despite the attendant grief.

Success in this realm seems to depend on several dimensions. The first of these is the ability, as one is present in the dying process, both to talk and to listen well. As we befriend death, it becomes increasingly easy to speak about this topic, to express our fears as well as our beliefs, and to be open and receptive to the thoughts and feelings of others. And the more we talk about it, the more comfortable we tend to become. To avoid the topic generally has the reverse effect as death remains a mysterious and frightening specter, one to be avoided at all cost. Moreover, when we avoid speaking about the topic with the dying person because of our own fears we may miss an opportunity to provide much needed and meaningful support in her or his final days of life.

Enjoying what is possible is the second dimension that may facilitate the process of dying well. Indeed, it is important that the entire focus not be on dying but, rather, that living out whatever time is available in the fullest way attainable be given equal time and attention. From attending to business to having fun, life continues to hold opportunities for many pleasures, both large and small. For example, all his adult life my father enjoyed having a cocktail before dinner. And even as he was in the final stages of dying, after he had lost all taste for food, he truly continued to savor a few tastes of his evening "libation" right up to the point at which he lost consciousness for the last time.

A third dimension to keep in mind is the blessing of messages both given and received. To be able to feel a sense of completion in the relationship with a dying loved one is a gift that goes a long way to ease our grief when death ultimately occurs. And when the pain of the loss can be somewhat assuaged by a message from "beyond the grave," everyone is the beneficiary. To illustrate, a client recently shared the story of a letter that was delivered to her by a friend 2 weeks after her husband died. In this letter, the dying man expressed gratitude for what he and his wife had shared together, apologies for presumed misdeeds, and wishes for his spouse to go on with her life and to find another partner with whom to share it. There is little doubt that the husband derived as much from the opportunity to send this letter as the wife did from receiving it.

The final issue is the importance of enabling the person who is terminally ill to die with dignity. Even in the final moments we must recognize the value of the dying person and honor the spirit that is now departing. For many this means providing a pain-free death in accord with the wishes of the one who is dying. For others, this may mean moving into the realm of euthanasia, which brings us to the subject of the next chapter.

THERAPEUTIC CONVERSATIONS
AND REFLECTIONS

∼

A terminally ill man in his early 70s had been battling a diagnosis of cancer for many years. However, the disease ultimately spread throughout his body and when it was determined that his life expectancy was less than 6 months, he and his wife agreed to make arrangements for in-home hospice care. Although the husband and wife were devoted to each other, the patient, "Fred," had always been the decision maker in the family and his wife, "Alice," had gladly deferred to him. They had three children, all of whom lived out of state and who also were busy with their own lives and growing families. These adult children were able to visit only infrequently and were unavailable for any further assistance. Alice, who was 10 years younger than Fred, was in good health, was quite willing to take on the role, and therefore became the designated caregiver, consistent as well with Fred's wishes.

(cont.)

Things went relatively smoothly during the initial stages of care. The hospice staff made routine visits, monitoring Fred's condition and Alice's well-being. Indeed, as long as Fred was able to be in charge of what was happening to him, Alice seemed to be quite capable of handling the demands of the situation. However, when Fred's condition began to deteriorate significantly, his authoritative style became more verbally abusive. He frequently vented his anger and frustration, both about his situation and his children's seeming lack of attention, on his wife, often refusing to do as she asked. Alice's response was to become upset and confused to the point where, finally, she was unable to make good decisions or follow through with the prescribed medical regimen.

The hospice staff worked hard in their efforts to support Alice, attempting to help her to understand Fred's reactions as normal and emphasizing the importance of providing the needed care despite his angry and abusive outbursts. However, these efforts were often undermined as the adult children, who were now calling often, gave conflicting suggestions and advice to their mother. They also complained to her about the way that the hospice staff were or were not handling various aspects of the situation despite the fact that they did not have firsthand knowledge about what was happening. This further confused Alice, who became less and less sure about what she should do.

The situation grew to crisis proportions when the hospice staff recommended that Fred be placed in a nursing home. Alice knew how important it had been for Fred to die at home. She also knew that she was not coping effectively. The adult children were not happy about this turn of events but made no effort to block the placement. However, Alice, who felt guilty about her inability to fulfill her husband's wishes, continued to vacillate about what to do, missing an opportunity to place him in the nursing home that was the family's first choice. By the time Fred finally was placed, Alice had sunk into a deep depression. The hospice staff was upset and feeling badly that things had not gone more favorably for the family, whose wishes they always attempted to support. Meanwhile, the adult children continued to be less than pleased.

As a family therapist reflecting on this scenario, I wonder whether a more satisfactory ending to similar situations might be achieved in the future if the initial assessment were to include a meeting with everyone involved—Alice, Fred, their three adult children and their spouses, relevant hospice staff, and medical team members. If the facilitation of such a meeting were beyond the purview of the hospice staff, I might consider recommending consultation with a professional trained to understand family systems and their dynamics as well as the impact of long-term illness, death, and grief.

I am aware that everyone has expertise that might truly help if it were respected and shared. Therefore, the goal of the proposed meeting would be to look realistically at the situation, to share information, to assess strengths, to make plans to shore up areas of potential weakness, and to provide for a meaningful and effective system of communication. For example, it might be appropriate to consider who else would be available to assist Alice and give her periodic respites from her care of Fred. It might be important for both Fred and Alice to articulate their expectations regarding contact with the children, whether by phone or in person. Additional significant information might be derived from understanding how in the past decisions generally were made in this family, what enabled them to handle other crises successfully, and where there were difficulties. It also would be crucial to spell out the specifics of the role of hospice staff members as well as the need for direct communication rather than succumbing to the temptation to engage in triangulation, for example, two people talking about a third person behind the back of the third person. And it would be important for the medical personnel to describe for everyone the typical course of the disease.

From my perspective, when death is anticipated there is great opportunity in the midst of crisis. When everyone is on board from the outset, when there is awareness of the complexities as well as the dynamics of the family and of their interactions with other systems, we may work together to support the goal of a peaceful dying and a good death.

CHAPTER 5

When the Question
of Euthanasia Emerges

∾

George Delury's Diary

New York, December 15, 1995: Following are excerpts from the computer
diary of George Delury, kept from February 27, 1994, until the death of his
wife, Myrna Lebov on July 4, 1994. The diary was released by District Attorney Robert M. Morgenthau of Manhattan following a grand jury investigation. Mr. Delury is now charged with manslaughter. [He eventually
pleaded guilty to attempted manslaughter and served 4 months of a 6-
month prison sentence.] Myrna had been a writer/editor but was stricken
with multiple sclerosis.

*February 27: Myrna's on the lower side of a downswing. It will get worse before
it gets better. She worries about every little thing, even denying the evidence of
the senses in order to express worry. Basically she wants reassurance. The big
thing tonight was the appointment with Petito [Ms. Lebov's doctor] tomorrow—
she wanted to pin down every detail in advance, including what he should recommend for her troubles, if he can recommend anything. She expressed special
concern about her incapacity to express herself well. It is unclear whether this is
an inability to hold onto a thought, an inability to find the words needed to express a thought, or both.*

*March 30: Nothing done. Myrna spent her time reading the paper and watching
the movie again. We talked in the evening, or rather, I talked. Myrna is more or
less rational. Able to see but not accept the reality of the situation. She is only
vaguely aware of the degree to which she is now adrift, with little autonomy left.*

She will admit in one moment that the situation is bad, that she can't write a book, that suicide might be the best solution, but moments later, it's as if nothing of this was said or was real. We can go through the same round again and again with no change. I doubt that anything will come of all this. The drift will get worse, until she's gone.

April 1: *It is now 11:30 P.M. Since 10:30 last night, I have had about 11 hours' sleep. I'm rested and it's good to have Myrna back for a bit. We talked some more about suicide and method today. She agreed to test a solution of cran juice and Elavil [an antidepressant] for taste and consistency tonight.*

Reviewing this memoir this evening, I was surprised that the last time we talked of suicide was only a month ago; it seemed much longer—probably a sign of the emotional roller coaster we're on.

May 1: *Sheer hell. Myrna is more or less euphoric. She spoke of writing a book today. She's interested in everything, wants everything explained and believes that every bit of bad news has some way out; e.g., our back tax bills: there must be something that can be done to make them less. She is encouraged in all this by her sister, Cleopatra, the Queen of Denial, who appears to believe that everything difficult here is my fault: Myrna's moods—the dysphoria is my fault, the euphoria is the good old Myrna; the Medicaid problem; the shortage of money, etc. It became an old-fashioned screaming match today, with me marching out saying I was going to get drunk. (Just a threat). When I came back, dry as ever, I told Myrna to tell Cleo that if she wishes to speak to me she will speak with respect or not at all.*

It's all just too much. I'm not going to come out of this in one piece or with any honor. I'm so tired of it all; maybe I should kill myself.

May 19: *My problem: if she asks for the poison now but seems very depressed, should I comply? Is she still autonomous? If I comply, I may be preserving my own interests more than hers. If I don't, she may be losing her last chance to make the decision. She's mentioned July 4 as "independence day," a possible suicide date, but at the rate her mind is deteriorating, she may not still be a whole, autonomous person by that time. I believe I will comply—on the rationale (rationalization?) that I will be saving her from a fate worse than death. (What an ironic cliché in this context!)*

July 3: *3:30 P.M. Myrna has pushed up the schedule to tonight. She seems mostly concerned about whether she can keep the amitriptyline [generic name for Elavil] down and whether it will work. She told me that when she set up her* pills on Saturday night, she only set them as far as Tuesday. She noted that future appointments had been made with the VN [visiting nurse] and she worries that the whole business may get me in trouble. She says she's spoken to both Alison [Ms. Lebov's niece] and Anne Tarpey [social worker] about her distaste for her severe functions, specifically the four caths a day. She was going to try to work on her suicide note, but at the last minute decided to watch "Forrest Gump" instead.

7:30 P.M. Myrna is now questioning the efficacy of the solution, a sure sign that she will not take it tonight and doesn't want to. So, confusion and hesitation strike again. If she changes her mind tonight and does decide to go ahead, I will be surprised.

July 4: 12:30 A.M. Myrna has just consumed about 3,000 to 4,000 mg. of the amitriptyline. Her courage was remarkable. Once begun, she went ahead as long as she could before it began to threaten the heaves. About 14 oz. of liquid, about half of what I had prepared. She said very little. Very direct and business-like. No tearful goodbyes, no jokes, just a let's-get-this-done approach. All rather anticlimactic.

Before we cathed and she took the solution, she expressed regret that she couldn't write letters to Beverly [Ms. Lebov's sister] and Alison. I said, Leave a message with me. She said, as if dictating, "I love you both very much. Please don't feel hurt; I know you did all you could for me. I'm bored with my bodily functions and my mind is going. It's better to end it now, while I can still do something."

We sat together on the bed for about a half-hour. She's soundly asleep now. I'll check back in about an hour.

I'm disappointed that she [was] finally so direct and single-minded about it. I wish she had said goodbye. I think there was an element of desperation there that simply blocked out everything else—the kind of total focus she used to have when she was writing.

2:15 A.M. Myrna is sleeping very soundly, breathing heavily. I'm going to grab an hour's sleep.

5:30 A.M. Slept through the alarm. It's over. Myrna is dead. Desolation.

[In his final entry, Mr. Delury noted that he called 911 at 8:20 A.M.]

—Taken from the Internet

When questions and concerns related to the topic of euthanasia arise, those searching for answers and resolution are plunged into the realms not only of medicine, public policy, and the law but also of ethics, morality, philosophy, religion, and spirituality (Becvar, 2000a). What is perhaps more significant, however, is that given the sensitive nature of this subject, searchers also are likely to be confronted with all the complexities of human relationships in the context of controversy, conflict, pain, and grief. Along with the various ethical, legal, and philosophical issues, what they tap into are deeply held feelings and beliefs regarding such issues as the meaning of life and death, the rights of individuals to make decisions for themselves, personal and professional perspectives on pain, suffering, treatment and cure, and the provision of care for the dying person that is considered to be adequate.

Fundamentally, euthanasia is about the right of a terminally ill person to determine how and when her or his death will occur. However, as the concept has been debated and dealt with pragmatically, a variety of permutations in meaning have emerged. For example, according to the Netherlands State Commission on Euthanasia, the term "euthanasia" refers to "the intentional termination of life by another party at the request of the person concerned" ("Final Report," 1987, p. 166) whereas assisted suicide is defined as "intentionally helping a patient to terminate his or her life at his or her request" (Scheper & Duursma, 1994, p. 4). In both cases assistance is provided to the dying person by someone else. However, a distinction is made between whether it is, as in the former instance, the other person, or, as in the latter instance, the dying person who actually implements the agreed on plan to end life.

Within the medical establishment three other distinctions relative to euthanasia also have been made. Voluntary active euthanasia (VAE) applies to those situations in which it is the physician who, at the request of the patient, gives a medication or somehow intervenes in such as manner as to cause death. Physician-assisted suicide (PAS) describes instances in which the physician provides information, resources, or direct assistance but it is the patient who terminates her or his own life (Watts, 1992). Finally, physician aid-in-dying refers to the discontinuation of treatment by the physician at the request of the patient (Celocruz, 1992).

Despite the recent resurgence of controversy, it is interesting to note that the debate around euthanasia is hardly a new one. The first euthanasia bill was drafted in Ohio, in 1906, and to greater and lesser degrees the topic has been the subject of public discussion not only in this country but also throughout the world since that time (Humphrey & Clement, 2000).

However, it was the phenomenal growth of medical technology and the related ability to extend life dramatically which brought the issue to the forefront of public attention during the 1990s. And in January 1997, the issue culminated with the decision of the U.S. Supreme Court to address the question "whether the Constitution gives terminally ill people a right to commit suicide with a doctor's help, or whether the government's stake to protect life is strong enough to outweigh whatever individual right may exist" ("Before the Court," 1997, p. 4E).

Following extensive debate relative to the cases in question, *Washington v. Glucksberg* and *Quill v. Vaco*, the Supreme Court ultimately ruled that laws banning physician assisted suicide do not violate either the U.S. Constitution or the equal protection clause of the Fourteenth Amendment. That is, individual states may, if they desire, choose to prohibit PAS. However, questions regarding the right of individual states to enact legislation permitting PAS remained undecided following the Court's decision (Brodeur, 1997). To explain:

> the court also validated the concept of "double effect," openly acknowledging that death hastened by increased palliative measures does not constitute prohibited conduct so long as the intent is the relief of pain and suffering. The majority opinion ended with the pronouncement that "Throughout the nation, Americans are engaged in an earnest and profound debate about the morality, legality and practicality of physician-assisted suicide. Our holding permits this debate to continue, as it should in a democratic society." (Humphrey & Clement, 2000, p. 373)

Even as this public debate continues, as no doubt it will for quite some time, on the private level those who are dying, as well as those who desire to support them, often find themselves having to come to conclusions and make decisions whose consequences cannot be predicted with certainty when the question of euthanasia emerges. They may be torn by a commitment, on the one hand, to honor the wishes of a loved one not to have to die in pain as well as an honest desire to alleviate that person's suffering. On the other hand, the choice of euthanasia may violate their own personal standards. In addition, they are aware of the risks involved, some of which may jeopardize their own well-being should they agree to participate in some form of euthanasia. For example, George Delury, whose journal excerpts provided the introduction to this chapter, and who was clearly implicated, pleaded guilty to the charge of having assisted his wife's suicide. Although prior to 1996 no one in the United States had been jailed for similar behavior, Delury was given a 6-month prison sentence (Humphrey & Clement, 2000).

At the same time, a variety of options, many of them within the bounds of the law and also aimed at providing comfort for and alleviating the suffering of the dying, certainly do exist. In this chapter I therefore begin with a consideration of legal issues related to euthanasia, looking first at what the general public needs to know and then at additional concerns about which professionals also should be aware. I next examine the various medical alternatives available to dying persons and their families, including a closer look at advance directives and hospice care. This discussion is followed by a consideration of religious and spiritual factors requiring attention relative to the right-to-die movement and choices within it. Finally, I conclude with a focus on family dynamics and the search both for workable compromises and, when appropriate, for professional assistance in dealing with conflict in the context of euthanasia questions.

LEGAL ISSUES

If we look back first at where other countries stand, we find that since 1984, the Netherlands has legalized both voluntary euthanasia and PAS. In Switzerland, assisted suicide has been allowed since 1937 and euthanasia is now permitted there as well. Although rarely practiced, voluntary euthanasia also is allowable in both Japan and Colombia (Humphrey & Clement, 2000).

As we shift our focus to the United States, we learn that Oregon is the only state that allows PAS. Although none of the states prohibits either suicide or attempted suicide, 36 states have statutes that explicitly make assisted suicide a criminal act; 7 states make assisted suicide a criminal act through the common law; and in six states the law concerning the legality of assisted suicide is unclear (Hemlock Society, 1997). Thus, the first order of business for anyone considering some form of euthanasia is to ascertain the law of the particular locality in which he or she resides.

In addition to knowing the laws relative to euthanasia, it also is important to be aware that according to the Supreme Court, there are two constitutionally permissible means of alleviating pain for dying persons when all other methods fail. As many may not understand, these methods ultimately will lead to the death of the person who is treated by either one: "The first is the 'morphine drip'—a continuous administration of morphine at a dose that will abolish pain. If that's not effective, a physician can also legally prescribe 'terminal sedation': barbiturates or other drugs providing continuous anesthesia. In the absence of feeding, death comes quickly" (Preston, 2000, p. 82).

The mechanism for becoming a candidate for these and other pain-alleviating procedures is an advance directive that is prepared in compliance with state law and is legally witnessed or notarized (Preston, 2000). Once again, however, it is important to be aware that states vary in terms of what is required and/or recognized. For example, California was the first state to enact legislation acknowledging the validity of advance directives. Passed in 1976, the California Natural Death Act permits individuals, in specific situations, to make prior plans for treatment at the end of life (Choice in Dying, 1991). Not only does this statute legally sanction advance directives, it also "protects physicians from being sued for failing to treat incurable illnesses" (Humphrey & Clement, 2000, p. 368). Today, many other states also have enacted living-will statutes as well as legislation that deals with procedures whose goal is to prolong life (Lush, 1993).

Along with the legalities relative to each state with which those who are critically ill must deal, professionals working in this arena also must be sensitive to several additional considerations. That is, marriage and family therapists have been advised to seek legal consultation regarding the laws of their state before attempting to work in any way with clients on issues related to euthanasia (Daw, 1996). Indeed, the degree to which it is permissible even to provide information must be clarified as does the extent to which a legal risk may be incurred just by virtue of having knowledge that a client intends to hasten her or his death. Further, should a marriage and family therapist be found guilty of compliance in a case involving assisted suicide, she or he would be considered in violation of the Code of Ethics of the American Association for Marriage and Family Therapy (2001) as well as, potentially, state licensure laws.

Within the social work profession, euthanasia has been determined by some to be unethical (e.g., Callahan, 1994), a conclusion based on various research studies which indicate that the judgment of most suicidal people is impaired as a function of some form of mental illness, particularly depression. Although "rational" suicide may exist, it is deemed to be a rare occurrence. In addition, social workers have expressed concern that legalized assisted suicide may lead to an increase in the rate of suicide in the general public, especially among young people, as the idea catches on and a stigma no longer is associated with it.

Psychologists appear to be divided in their opinions regarding the legalization of assisted suicide. For one group, which takes a position similar to that of social workers, the desire for assisted suicide is viewed as a symptom of mental illness. For another group, a supportive position is taken based on the belief "that suicide can be a rational act and that psychologists and other mental-health professionals should be allowed to help such patients without fear of legal or professional repercussions" (Clay, 1997, p. 1). Consistent with this lack of consensus, the American Psychological Association does not take a position either for or against assisted suicide. However, quality of care at the end of life and informed decision making which reflects correct and complete assessment of the patient certainly are supported (Farberman, 1997).

Professional counselors have been advised to be prepared to work with clients who may be considering some form of euthanasia (Kiser, 1996). At the same time, it has been noted that a reevaluation of standards may be required to avoid violating the ethical guidelines established by the American Counseling Association. Indeed, regardless of differences in professional affiliation, the recommendation to be well informed and to take precautions to avoid violation of either the law or codes of ethics is consistent for all who work in this area. In addition, along with knowledge relative to the legal arena, it also is important for mental health professionals to be familiar with the various issues that may arise within the medical realm.

MEDICAL ISSUES

Information and knowledge about the various treatment options as well as about what the choices regarding specific medical interventions actually may mean are essential for anyone making decisions relative to the final stage of life. It is important that those who are dying, along with family members and other support persons, be aware of steps that may be taken to ensure that the desired end-of-life care actually takes place. For example, according to the federal Patient Self-Determination Act (PSDA), a part of the 1990 Omnibus Budget and Reconciliation Act which went into effect in December 1991, health care providers (mainly hospitals, nursing homes and home health agencies) are required to give patients information about their rights under state law to make advance directives. States are permitted to specify the actual content of their laws with reference to advance directives, but the PSDA also requires that providers have written institutional policies relative to advance directives and that they document whether or not an advance directive has been executed by the patient (Choice in Dying, 1991). Indeed, advance directives "are becoming an increasingly important component of medical decision making for incompetent patients" (McCrary & Botkin, 1989, p. 2411).

Unfortunately, however, as patients and their families attempt to create advance directives, they may not fully understand the ramifications of various choices. They also may be unaware of the options that actually are available, or may only become aware at the point of crisis, when decision making is much more challenging. For example, in regard to treatment choices, resuscitation procedures performed following cardiac arrest may maintain life, but they also may be severely debilitating, particularly for the frail elderly. Such knowledge is not widely held unless one is part of the medical profession and it is certainly inconsistent with what is portrayed in TV shows. There also may be a lack of awareness that the kind of pain medications described in the previous section are legally available. In addition, patients may not realize that without unanimity among family members, the plan they have created in advance may be negated, thus preventing adherence to their expressed wishes (Preston, 2000).

To illustrate the dilemma, let us consider an 88-year-old patient who suffered from chronic obstructive pulmonary disease. Following many hospitalizations, the patient specifically requested not to have any more invasive procedures, such as a bronchoscopy, during which a tube is inserted into the lungs to drain fluid that impedes respiration. When pneumonia recurred and the patient was once again hospitalized, the physician informed family members that unless a bronchoscopy was performed, the patient would literally drown as a result of fluid in the lungs. The eldest child, who had the power of attorney to make such decisions, was unable to allow this parent simply to die under such circumstances. Thus this child gave permission for the procedure, which was performed, and ultimately the patient lived for several more months. In this case, no family members disputed the decision. Nevertheless, it clearly illustrates the way in which the wishes of the dying person may be overridden when there is not total agreement or when the burden of responsibility for decision making feels too great.

Keeping such provisos in mind, advance directives may be designed in the form of either a living will or a health care proxy. A living will is a document created by a competent adult in which she or he delineates specific instructions related to medical treatment in the event that she or he should become incapacitated at some time in the future. The document becomes a will by virtue of the inclusion of these directions. It is designated a living will because it is intended to go into effect prior to the death of the person (Annas, 1991, p. 1210).

A health care proxy is created by means of a durable power of attorney. In this case the competent adult designates an agent who is charged with making health care and treatment decisions in the event that she or he should become unable to make such decisions at some time in the future. As in the illustration presented previously, however, it is noteworthy that there is evidence suggesting a lack of fit between what patients would have chosen and what others ultimately choose for them (Lambert, Gibson, & Nathanson, 1990). In terms of the validity of this alternative, however, although existing laws regarding the assignment of a durable power of attorney may be sufficient, many states have enacted additional legislation regarding proxy designation relative to health care (Annas, 1991).

There are also two options for the focus of an advance directive, including either the clinical condition or the values history (Doukas & McCullough, 1991; McLean, 1994). When the advance directive focuses on the clinical condition, the specific circumstances under which the person would or would not want to live are specified. In other words, consideration is given to specific medical decisions that are to be made should the person be unable to express his or her wishes when the time comes.

When the advance directive focuses on the values history, the circumstances under which life is not preferred, even when further medical treatment is available, are specified. In this case, consideration is given to the assumptions and decision-making processes used by the person now and on the basis of which future medical determinations are to be made. Indeed, a reason for selecting this option is that "while we cannot predict our future, we can at least explain ourselves now. The explanation may help ensure that the person we are, and hope to be, is respected by others who must stand in our stead" (Lambert, Gibson, & Nathanson, 1990, p. 211).

Regardless of the form selected, it is crucial that in the process of creating advance directives the person be competent, be able to understand what he or she is doing, execute the directive voluntarily, be fully informed regarding all ramifications, and, ultimately, give his or her consent for its implementation (Beauchamp & Childress, 1994). Those involved with supporting this process also must be sensitive to ethnic and cultural variations and values regarding, for example, autonomy and the right to make decisions (Young & Jex, 1992), which in some cases rests with the individual and in others with the family as a whole. Documents so created also must be internally consistent and must include only those dimensions within the scope of standard medical practice (VA Medical Center, 1993).

As useful as advance directives may be when the time comes to refer to them, an equally important aspect of their creation may be "the process individuals go through defining what quality of life means to them by specifying their values and beliefs to their families and physicians before they face a crisis situation" (Hoffman, 1994, p. 229). What is more, through the use of narrative methods and story-based assessments (Kielstein & Sass, 1993), more sensitive interactions between patients and physicians may be encouraged as professionals are challenged to integrate various value positions into clinical practice. Finally, the creation of an advance directive may enable the dying person to retain a sense of control even in the face of the inevitable and ultimate loss of control that death represents. Having the knowledge that one will receive only the treatment that is consistent with one's own choices and/or the values according to which one has lived may indeed be a powerful source of comfort.

According to some, if the goal of the dying person truly is to experience comfort at the end of life, the best option is hospice care (Preston, 2000). Hospice programs are designed for those with a terminal diagnosis, regardless of the particular disease or condition with which they may be dealing. They use a team approach and generally include physicians, nurses, and social workers. Hospice care may be provided either in a designated facility or in the home of the dying person. In the latter case, a primary support person usually must be designated and available in order to qualify for services. Hospice care thus represents a holistic approach, one that recognizes the following:

> Of the fundamental needs of persons as they die, only the need to control physical symptoms is uniquely medical. Their more basic needs are broader than the scope of medicine. They need shelter from the elements, a place to be. They need help with personal hygiene and assistance with elimination. They need nourishment or, as death comes close, sips of fluid to moisten their mouth and throat. They need companionship, and they need others to recognize their continued existence. (Byock, 1997, p. 247)

One of the basic assumptions on which the hospice movement has been built is that relief of physical pain is always possible. However, there may be a lack of knowledge about and/or a lack of availability of this type of care given the relatively recent appearance of hospice programs in this country. In addition, some may feel that the only acceptable option in the face of inevitable deterioration or intractable pain is some form of euthanasia. Indeed, those who advocate for legalizing PAS generally believe that it is the most humane response, one that not only allows an individual to die with dignity (Hemlock Society, 1997; McLean, 1996; Weir, 1992) but also is respectful of life (Dworkin, 1993). Others argue that euthanasia is totally unacceptable, is demeaning of life, and represents an option whose impact will be to undermine one of the most basic tenets of our moral code, that which prohibits causing the death of another person (Beauchamp & Childress, 1994). Such issues and considerations, of course, move us into the realm of religion and spirituality, one which also certainly deserves attention in the context of questions that may emerge relative to euthanasia.

RELIGIOUS AND SPIRITUAL ISSUES

According to religious scholar Philip Kapleau (1989), over the course of history institutionalized religions "have taken every conceivable view of suicide, from recommending it to resolutely and uncompromisingly opposing it" (p. 130). Noting that often there has been no differentiation between suicide and euthanasia, Kapleau provides as examples those cultures in which it was simply presumed that the death of husbands or masters would be followed by the suicide of wives and servants. On the other hand, he cites St. Augustine, for whom suicide was considered to be a crime both because the possibility of repentance is precluded and because, as a form of homicide, it violates the biblical sixth commandment against killing. In Kapleau's opinion, both Orthodox Protestantism and Judaism also have been forceful in their repudiation of self-destruction.

At the same, there often is lack of agreement about the stance of particular religious belief systems toward suicide and euthanasia, depending on the perspective of the observer. Thus, for example, Buddhism has been described as both supportive (Perrett, 1966) and hostile (Kapleau, 1989; Keown & Keown, 1995) to this act. And certainly there are members of a variety of other traditions who, although sharing similar religious beliefs in general, would position themselves on either side of this specific issue.

Currently in our society, some of the most steadfast opposition to efforts to legalize euthanasia is coming from religious institutions. At the same time, it is interesting to note the following:

> Most Christian and Jewish groups approve of the withholding and withdraw-
> ing of life-sustaining treatment, as do most Eastern religions, although the
> latter are less specific about it. Allowing a hopelessly ill person to die by not
> introducing medical technology is widely accepted today by a broad range of
> faiths. Only Mormons, Evangelicals, and other strict Gospel denominations
> are opposed to this practice in the West, while Islam is opposed in the East.
> (Humphrey & Clement, 2000, p. 186)

Ultimately, of course, each person must reconcile her or his own moral/ethical position with the values and standards of the particular tradition to which she or he makes recourse. Another aspect of the dilemma, however, resides in the extent to which various traditions either assume responsibility for such choices or understand that personal choice takes precedence. What is more, even those who do not subscribe to a particular faith system have values and core beliefs that must be taken into consideration and also must be reconciled.

For example, from a spiritual orientation that is inclusive of traditions that may or may not be derived from a particular religious belief system (Becvar, 1996), questions about what is most appropriate, rather than what is right or wrong, at the level of the individual soul may require attention. Indeed, we might even consider the notion, or at least the possibility, that it is we who have participated in creating our particular life circumstances, including when and how we will die, and that to negate them in any way may preclude an opportunity for soul growth (Becvar, 1997). We also may wish to consider the possibility that despite motives based on compassion, participation in ending life may not be the "most loving response" (Becvar, 2000a).

Clearly, this is an area of focus that is fraught with challenges. Indeed, we might do well to remind ourselves of the old adage advising against engaging in conversations about politics or religion. Such advice is based on the awareness of the importance given to opinions and ideas in these two areas. Some of the most basic assumptions according to which we live our lives are to be found in or are expressed within the context of our particular religious and/or political orientation.

Relative to euthanasia questions, it is inevitable that moral ideas and values derived from various religious and spiritual belief systems not only will come into play but also often will be challenged as family members search for answers and seek to make the best decisions possible. Attempts to come to terms with and resolve differences must take place even as sincere efforts are made both to support the dying person and to manage grief. Given the complexity of the circumstances and depending upon how such issues are handled, the family is at great risk for being torn apart as a function of irreconcilable differences. It therefore behooves us to take a closer look both at family dynamics and at ways in which professionals may be a useful resource at the end of life.

FAMILY DYNAMICS AND INTERVENTIONS

Dealing with end-of-life issues is inherently and inevitably stressful and challenging. Under even the most benign circumstances, the dying person and his or her family members, friends, and professional caregivers come face to face with the mortality that is a fundamental yet often denied aspect of human life. Fear, grief, and pain, as well as a variety of related emotions, become constant companions. Old angers and hurts may surface as there is recognition that time is running out. What is more, even the desire to be supportive and to do what one truly believes is in the best interests of the dying person does not preclude the probability of discord and controversy. Whether the person who is dying is a child, a young adult, middle age, or elderly, there may be both internal conflict and external disagreement among family members about how best to proceed.

For example, we need only think about decisions around long-term care for aging parents. Although placement in a retirement facility may seem the best or perhaps the only viable option, the daughters and sons who must make such decisions may experience a host of mixed reactions. They may feel guilty about not being able to care for their parents in their own home, may have to struggle financially to make such a placement possible, may be angered by the responsibility, may be relieved that adequate care is being provided, and may be sad about what such a decision connotes. Further, siblings may disagree about what are the best choices for their parents. Some may feel overburdened when there is perceived to be a lack of participation by others.

If one adds to this kind of context, one that contains all the ingredients guaranteed to produce a high level of emotionality, the dimension of euthanasia, we produce a recipe for extremely volatile human interaction and family dynamics. To illustrate, in a made-for-TV movie entitled, *A Time to Die*, we first meet a family in which the four children are all grown and have begun the process of establishing careers and creating families of their own. The parents have maintained a long-term and very loving marriage. The mother has not worked outside the home and has focused most of her energies on her husband and children. The father is a well-respected surgeon who works hard but also enjoys the benefits of financial success. There is a low level of discord between various family members, including some sibling rivalry as well as parent–child conflicts and tensions. Basically, however, the family is portrayed as healthy but also having both many normal foibles and lots of positive interaction.

Problems arise when the father is diagnosed with Alzheimer's disease. Not only does this mean the end of his career, it also portends the kind of death he saw his own mother experience, one he has promised he will never go through himself. Early on in the course of the disease he therefore enlists the support of his wife to help him end his life when the time comes that he can no longer manage for himself. In the midst of her grief about her husband's impending debilitation, the wife is now confronted with his request to help him die. At first horrified, she ultimately agrees to support her husband and his choice. However, what appears to be irreparable damage is done to the family once the children learn about their parents' decision.

One of the children is ambivalent but agrees to help the mother. Two of the children keep their distance. The other child is vehemently opposed based on religious convictions and abhorrence for the idea of euthanasia. Ultimately, in the midst of raging court battles, the father is kidnapped by one of his children. He then is placed in a residential facility, the mother is denied access to her husband, various siblings won't speak to each other, and huge sums of money are required to meet legal fees. Although this is a fictional account, it certainly depicts a potentially valid scenario, one worthy of consideration relative to euthanasia questions.

When dealing with end-of-life issues, and particularly euthanasia considerations, the wisest course of action would probably include a search for professional advice and assistance. A third party, one who is less involved emotionally and especially one who is comfortable working in this realm, might provide a more stable context within which to consider issues and options. For professionals so engaged, having determined the limits of legal and ethical liability, a primary focus would be the exploration of potential choices and their possible ramifications. First, however, there must be a careful assessment of the dying person and his or her ability to make a competent and autonomous decision. Accordingly, it is suggested (Battin, 1994) that questions such as the following should be considered before proceeding:

1. Is the person making a request for help? For example, when somebody wants assistance in suicide is it in fact cloaking some other aspect or some other solution which may be found?

2. Why is the person consulting a physician or mental health professional? Has the consultation been sought because the person has certain expectations from the professionals?

3. What has kept the person from attempting or committing suicide so far? Is it fear of consequences, or given advanced illness or physical limitations they simply cannot obtain the means of causing death? Is the time for suicide not yet right? Or is the person seeking some sort of approval?

4. Is there quest for help in suicide a request for someone else to decide?

5. How stable is the request? Has this been part of a long term decision, or a short term response as a result of some traumatic event, e.g., diagnosis of serious illness, death of a friend or relative? Also, when the person thinks of suicide, does someone else come to mind? Does the person frequently change his or her mind about suicide?

6. Is the request consistent with a person's basic values? If there is a discrepancy, can the discrepancy be justified?

7. How far in the future would the suicide take place? Is it intended to solve a future problem, the eventual onset of intractable pain or mental deterioration, or to put an end to problems currently occurring?

8. Are the medical facts cited in the request accurate?

9. How accurate are the other non-medical facts cited in the request, for example, that others who assist in an attempt may be subject to criminal penalties, life insurance coverage, etc.?

10. Is the suicide plan financially motivated? Is it intended to avoid catastrophic medical expenses?

11. Has the person considered the effect of his or her suicide on other persons, also the stigma associated with suicide?

12. Does the person fear becoming a burden? Is he or she being manipulated by family members, etc., or has there been frank and open communication between the person and their loved ones?

13. What cultural influences are shaping the person's choice? Are religious beliefs, prejudices especially against the handicapped and aged contributing to a feeling of worthlessness?

14. Are the person's affairs in order?

15. Has the person picked a method of committing suicide? Does the person know what kinds of injuries are likely to result if the attempt is not fatal? Does the person want to stick to this one method only? If the person hasn't chosen one method does this make them ambivalent about committing suicide at all or is it simply lack of information?

16. Would the person be willing to tell others about his or her suicide plans?
17. Does the person see suicide as the only way out? (Becvar, 2000a, pp. 453–454)

In addition, there also must be concern both for the deeply held beliefs and values of family members as well for the relationship issues that may come into play. One important area of exploration might be that of individual beliefs about who has the right to make a decision about ending life and what such a decision might mean for those who participate and/or survive. Similarly, individual stories about illness (Kleinman, 1988) as well as about the meaning of both life and death require attention. Perhaps most significant to the outcome of such a process will be the ability to deal with and somehow resolve various divergent positions espoused by family members as well as feelings of ambivalence different individuals may be experiencing.

Professionals working in this area thus are challenged to be knowledgeable, sensitive, and competent in their efforts to guide dying persons and their families through the turbulent waters created in the wake of euthanasia considerations. They also must recognize the limits of what is possible. That is, despite their best efforts, consensus may never be achieved and it may not be possible to prevent lasting damage to the family. Indeed, as they share this awareness, they may achieve a useful shift to a focus on relationships within the family.

Family members thus may be encouraged to speak about their relationships with each other, and particularly with the person who is dying. They may be invited to move beyond a concern with principles, however important, to reflections on the meaning for the relationship that a decision related to ending one's own life has. And as all family members are able to express their deep caring and concern as well as their pain and grief, some sense of resolution may be achieved.

THERAPEUTIC CONVERSATIONS AND REFLECTIONS

∿

Two young men, partners in a committed, homosexual relationship who had been together for many years, and who had lived with the reality of AIDS for half that time, recognized that for one of them the end was drawing near. They had discussed the possibility of creating a mutual suicide pact but had rejected it based both on their religious convictions and on concerns about the impact of such an act on the families in which they grew up. They also had briefly discussed, but had dismissed for similar reasons, the idea of having one assist the other in ending life when it became too unbearable. What they were looking for instead was a way to die with dignity and to avoid the horrors many of their friends had experienced in their AIDS-related dying processes.

Both young men were well educated and well informed. They also had a strong support system consisting of both friends and family members. And they were intent on changing the legacy often left by AIDS. That is, they wanted to model what might be possible in terms of alleviating suffering and using the fact of their impending deaths as a catalyst for self-understanding and growth.

Once it was clear what their goal was, the focus quickly turned to the potential utility for both men of creating advance directives, with a particular emphasis on the use of a values history. Having agreed that this was consistent with their desires, a series of deep, soul-searching conversations then ensued. Accordingly, family backgrounds and relationship histories were explored, important values and their sources or creation were articulated, and expectations and desires were described.

Each man was encouraged to keep a journal describing his process of discovery. Not only might this be helpful to the process, but one day it also might become part of a guide left to others who found themselves walking a similar path. And, as appropriate, each was invited to let significant family members and friends know how and when these others had played an important role in the development of their personal philosophies, especially, their moral and ethical value systems, and to thank them for their contributions and influence.

To be clear about what their medical options might be, the clients also were urged to read further regarding their legal rights and to consult with the physicians who might be caring for them in the final days and weeks of their life. In addition, they identified and talked with family members to ascertain their degree of willingness to provide care should either be too incapacitated to do so or, as now seemed likely, one survived the other.

(cont.)

Although both men loved life, neither feared death. They had seen so much of it and had lost so many friends that the idea of death had become familiar, almost a constant companion. Rather, it was the anticipation of pain and debilitation as well as concerns about becoming a burden that were most worrisome. And each was anxious about having to watch the other die an excruciating and demeaning death.

Once they had examined and articulated their values and beliefs, they were able to define in clear terms what would be considered an acceptable quality of life and the circumstances under which they would no longer wish to have life prolonged by extreme measures of any kind. Each also was able to designate a person who would act as a health care proxy and to have this choice formalized by means of a durable power of attorney. They also were able to share with all appropriate friends and family members the fruits of their explorations and decision-making processes and to secure from them assurance that their wishes would be followed. And they were able to celebrate together what they had created.

Having looked into the face of death and having learned from the experiences of others, these two men were able to fulfill several goals, more even than they had anticipated or desired at the outset. They certainly felt that they had learned and grown a great deal during the course of their conversations and explorations. They also experienced a measure of control in the face of a disease that seems literally to be out of control. They were able to anticipate and hopefully avoid problems that might hamper their desire to die well. They felt confident that they would receive the palliative care they desired and that their deaths would not be demeaning in any way. What is more, they had helped to bring their family and community members closer together, perhaps easing the grief they undoubtedly felt and would continue to experience. Perhaps most important, they had freed themselves up to be able to focus on life and living in the full knowledge and awareness of their death and dying. Indeed, they had succeeded in creating a significant legacy, one they hoped might prove to be of great value to others who find themselves facing similar realities and challenges.

CHAPTER 6

When a Child Dies

∽

All of my life I have been able to make positive interpretations out of the most tragic events, to find some good even in the darkest moments. For 2 weeks I have struggled to do this with the death of my son. I have decided, at least at this point, that there is absolutely nothing good about the fact that my son has died.

Each morning, before I am fully awake, I become aware of the reality that his living presence is no longer with us. Each morning I once again experience the terror and icy pain in my chest and arms that have been a nearly constant companion since the call came from the hospital. Each day I find myself struggling through mundane tasks until I reach a state of numbness that allows the burden to seem a little lighter. But in the evening I know the process will have to be repeated all over again come morning.

9/11

For years I have heard the expression that God doesn't give us a burden that we can't bear. While I certainly knew that this was no guarantee, I felt in my heart that I could not bear to lose one of my children. I did not think I could survive if anything happened to either of them. Well, I am surviving, so I was wrong. But I do not believe I will ever be able to get over my son's death. Hopefully, I will be able to find a way to come to terms with the reality so that I can do more than survive. An even greater hope is that I can someday feel that I have not really lost him, that somehow the incredible bond of love and respect we shared continues even beyond death.

Everything seems so wrong to me. One minute I have a strong, healthy, vital son who is doing nothing more harmful than training for triathlons. The next minute his body is so injured that I cannot recognize him. Healthy people shouldn't just die. I have never before seen a dead person and the first dead person I see is my child. Parents shouldn't outlive their children. A mother shouldn't be receiving the benefits of a life insurance policy from her son. It should be the other way around.

9/13

Three weeks today.

9/14

Too much pain, too many thoughts to write anything yesterday. I keep thinking that writing things down will help me sort things out. But some days even that is too much of an effort.

I seem to do everything at half-speed and doing anything requires a tremendous amount of concentration. I can get distracted sometimes for as much as an hour but I'm aware all the time of a repressed scream that wants to be voiced. I try and try to remember how it felt to go about the daily routines of life before all this happened.

I can't get it out of my mind that my son has just been snatched away from us. But this gets confused when I walk by his picture, which smiles back at me and he seems to be here with us just as he always was. I still believe that his spirit lives in and with us but it just isn't enough. And yet I know it has to be.

9/18

My feeling of terror in the morning has changed to listlessness and despair. I hate having to accept the reality all over again, and having to deal with the emptiness I feel. I want to keep sleeping in the hope that I will at least see my son in my dreams if I can't see him while I am awake. I keep waiting for him or for God to respond to me but I'm not even sure what or how to pray.

I keep trying to find times to be alone and quiet and just wait and listen. But that is hard because my head is in such a turmoil.

9/22

Yesterday was horrible. My worst day yet. One big giant step backward. I went to bed feeling afraid of the dark. I didn't sleep well and I woke early, still feeling afraid of the dark. I felt as though I was coming unglued. I felt that I simply could not live with my son's loss. My tears, which are never far from the surface, would not stop. Eventually I pulled myself together enough to get through the day but the pain and sadness I felt still persist.

9/26

I want this nightmare to end and I know it won't and I know the fact that I'm tired and I don't feel well isn't helping but sometimes the whole situation seems unbearable! I suppose mornings are so difficult because I wake up and realize that the nightmare isn't going to go away and that I have to go on in spite of it.

I'm aware of how much I'm bouncing emotionally and I know it's normal and I know that time is supposed to help but none of that matters very much because I simply can't stand the fact that my son died. I can't stand the fact that we are all miserable and there is nothing any of us can do to change what happened. Just 5 weeks ago we had it all: love, laughter, contentment at being exactly what and who we were. Not perfect, but enjoying each other and caring about each other. I used to tell my husband in the evening how good it felt to have everybody home at the end of our long, busy days. I loved to fix dinner for the kids and have them tease me about what I did or didn't make. Food was such an important part of my son's life and he was a joy to cook for because he appreciated it so much.

10/22

I look at my son's pictures and I still can't believe what happened. None of it makes sense. While I am able to do a better job of controlling my grief, it is always there just beneath the surface. The only bright spot is my belief that my son is fine. However, that certainly is not true for the rest of us. I long for my relationship with my son to be restored. I miss him. I miss the pure joy of seeing him thrive and grow. I miss the pleasure of his company. I cry because of the huge void I feel in myself and in my life.

When I talked to my daughter on the phone last evening I was very cheerful and I told her I was fine. I don't want her to worry about me and I want so badly for her to feel better. But I'm not fine and I wonder if she knows it just as she knows she is not fine. It is hard to imagine how we will ever be truly fine again.

Twelve years later

As I read through the journal written during the first days and weeks following my son's death I find myself reliving the pain as though it were just yesterday. Tears are my immediate response and all of the heaviness returns. And yet, for the most part, I really am fine again. My life has been forever changed and there is much for which I am truly grateful. The joy I now experience is in direct proportion to the deep grief which also is an integral part of my being. I no longer expect the grief to diminish—any more than I would like to see my joy decreased. What is different is that I have learned to live with the grief, to expand myself, to be able to accommodate simultaneously both sadness and happiness.

The sadness is very predictable and particularly evident each time we celebrate a holiday, an anniversary, a birthday, a special family occasion. At other times, it may catch me by surprise in the midst of the most routine activities. It may only be a fleeting awareness or a moment of wishful thinking. But in either case, my son's death is an experience that keeps on happening, time and time and time again. And I continue to miss him with all my heart as I know I always will.

However, the sadness no longer prevents me from living my life to the fullest. In fact, I now am able to understand and enjoy happiness in a way that probably was not available to me prior to my son's death. I value the small, precious moments, the sharing times with my family and friends, the quiet spaces for walking or meditation, the beauty of each day, as some of life's greatest gifts. My priorities have changed and I am unwilling to settle for situations which are compromising to the integrity of my being in any way. I also can make music again, something I never thought I would be able to do. I believe I have grown in my ability to be compassionate, to understand the pain that others may be experiencing. I have found a whole new way of thinking, working, of being, one that enables me to trust that all the events in my life somehow make sense. Above all, I know that my relationship with my son continues, that nothing can break the connection of love we share. And I can say with all sincerity that despite the pain, I give thanks for the growth that was triggered by his death.

—DSB

An examination of the history of family life in Western society reveals that attitudes toward children, including the idea of childhood, have been subject to dramatic changes over time. For example, until as recently as 300 years ago, what has been described as "a feeling of indifference toward a too-fragile childhood" (Aries, 1962, p. 39) tended to be the norm. That is, given the state of medical knowledge as well as other harsh realities of earlier times, parents could anticipate that few if any of their offspring would survive into adulthood. What is more, there seems to have been a general lack of recognition that an infant had either mental abilities or a definitive personality. However, throughout the 14th, 15th, and 16th centuries a gradual evolution apparently occurred. Accordingly,

> although demographic conditions did not greatly change between the thirteenth and seventeenth centuries, and although child mortality remained at a very high level, a new sensibility granted these fragile, threatened creatures a characteristic which the world had hitherto failed to recognize in them: as if it were only then that the common conscience had discovered that the child's soul too was immortal. (Aries, 1962, p. 43)

Such a change in perception regarding the nature of the child, attributed in large part to the growing influence of Christianity (Aries, 1962), was made manifest particularly through artwork. Thus, for the first time we begin to find portraits of children by themselves and family paintings arranged around children, who were central to the composition. Also significant was that children no longer were portrayed as little adults but now wore clothing distinctive to their age group.

During this period, family life became more private and the use of nicknames, or terms of endearment, began to emerge. There also was a greater concern for the general health and well-being of family members. Thus, by the 18th century, it could be said that "nobody would now dare to seek consolation for losing a child in the hope of having another, as parents could have admitted doing only a century before. The child was irreplaceable, his death irreparable" (Aries, 1962, p. 401). Such sentiments, of course, continue today, as families focus primarily on the rearing and supporting of children, and the death of a child is universally acknowledged to be one of life's worst tragedies (Gilbert, 1997).

Indeed, the loss of a child generally is experienced by parents as pushing them almost "beyond endurance" (Knapp, 1986) as they struggle to come to terms with an event that in our era seems almost inconceivable. For, as the rate of infant mortality decreases and life expectancy increases, we often allow ourselves to be lulled into the belief that everyone who is born not only will survive but also will live to a ripe old age. We tend to anticipate that events will unfold in a neat and orderly fashion, and that certainly the young will outlive the old:

The sun rises in the east. Winter inevitably yields to spring. The tides ebb and flow with comforting predictability. Seeds take root, push their greenery toward the sun, bloom, produce new seed, wither, and die, all in orderly progression according to nature's plan. When an aged parent dies, though we may grieve deeply for the personal loss, the world is not turned upside down. Nature's plan, the predictability of the universe, remains intact. When a child dies, the very ground on which we depend for stability heaves and quakes and the rightness and orderliness of our existence are destroyed. Nothing in life prepares us; no coping skills were learned. Parents who lose children are thrown into chaos. The loss of a child is shattering, unique among losses. (J. R. Bernstein, 1997, p. 3)

Unfortunately, and however unprepared we may be, the truth is that people do die at every age and life is not necessarily neat and orderly. Further, although mortality rates certainly have improved or at least maintained in recent years, childhood deaths, caused by both illness and accidents, continue to occur in all age categories. Table 6.1 presents a look at childhood death rates from 1985 to 1995.

In addition, whereas Table 6.1 depicts only childhood deaths, it is also important to remember that regardless of age, when a son or daughter dies, the parents experience the loss of a child. Certainly the mourning process varies greatly as a function of the different kinds of relationships parents have with children at different ages and stages of life. However, no evidence exists that suggests that the loss of a child is any more or less devastating depending on the age or time at which his or her death occurs (Rando, 1988).

Further, although often ignored or denied, such an assessment also

TABLE 6.1. Childhood Death Rates from All Causes

	Deaths per 1,000 population						
	1985	1990	1991	1992	1993	1994	1995
Under 1 year	10.6	9.2	8.9	8.5	8.4	8.0	7.6
1–4 years	0.5	0.5	0.5	0.4	0.4	0.4	0.4
5–9 years	0.2	0.2	0.2	0.2	0.2	0.2	0.2
10–14 years	0.3	0.3	0.3	0.2	0.3	0.3	0.3
15–19 years	0.8	0.9	0.9	0.8	0.9	0.9	0.8

Internet sources: Centers for Disease Control and Prevention, National Center for Health Statistics.

may be applicable to the loss of a child during pregnancy (Speckhard, 1997). Although all parents who lose a child experience the destruction of their hopes, dreams, and expectations for that child, there is a kind of cultural disenfranchisement of loss during pregnancy. That is, there is generally less acknowledgment of the loss and the pain it entails. Among other things, what this means for parents who experience a miscarriage or still-birth is less support than is generally available for those who have lost a child following a live birth.

In every case, the grief experienced at the death of a child has been described as unique, given the special bond and distinctive relationship that exists between parents and their children (Klass, 1988). Compromised by such a loss is the sense of identity derived from being a parent, as well as the various interconnections with others which exist as a function of this relationship. Not only is the parental bond severed, so also is the child-focused interaction with grandparents or potential grandparents. And in the case of the death of an older child, relationships with his or her friends and their parents also are likely to be severely altered.

In addition, parents generally feel not only a tremendous sense of obligation but also a deep commitment to care for and safeguard their children. When a child dies there is a feeling of somehow having failed in this regard, despite the lack of any culpability. Finally, perceptions regarding the unfairness of the experience add enormously to the grief experienced by parents who lose a child.

Although the idea of helping grieving parents might therefore seem to present an insurmountable challenge, there is much that can be offered by way of support. Accordingly, this chapter, first of all, considers the importance of stories. This consideration includes the need many parents feel to talk about their experience and thus for there to be others willing to listen. It also includes the need parents may feel to find or create a story that will enable them, somehow, to make meaning of an event that has thrown their world into total disarray. Second, the chapter focuses on differences in grieving styles and the conflict that may be engendered between parents as each engages both in a personal struggle to come to terms with the loss and an attempt to be supportive of the other. Our third concern is that of finding ways to help grieving parents respond to other children so that further damage to the family as a result of one child's death may be avoided. The fourth section focuses on parents who have lost a child either during pregnancy or in the days immediately following the child's birth. Finally, the chapter concludes with some thoughts about the ways life may be forever changed when a child dies.

THE IMPORTANCE OF STORIES

When working with or seeking to help parents who have lost a child, one of the most important factors of which to be aware is the need they generally feel to be able to talk about what has happened (J. R. Bernstein, 1997; Knapp, 1986). Indeed, as noted by one bereaved parent, "The most essential ingredient, in fact, in surviving well—besides facing reality—is to speak of the dead child unashamedly" (Schiff, 1977, p. 101). And being able to speak unashamedly means that the parents can tell their story without feeling that others will be put off by the expression of their grief or that they can't handle it. Without a willing ear, someone who is able to listen to, and perhaps cry with, the grieving parent, that parent experiences something akin to denial, as if the child never lived, the death didn't occur, the pain is not real. Further, as described by a mother who lost both of her young children in an automobile accident, the need to tell one's story generally continues long after the death:

> The working class, immigrants, the self-taught cranks, the handicapped, the unemployed and grieving parents are more alike than people think. They have at least one thing in common: they have to make Herculean efforts to hold a normal, banal, bouncy conversation. They can think of only one thing: the moment when they might introduce a sentence about their misfortune. Thirteen years have passed, and I still cannot last half a day without evoking my daughters. (Jurgensen, 1999, p. 147)

In addition to being able to tell their story, and to do so as often as seems necessary, parents also need to be able to speak of or make reference to the dead child and events in his or her life. The tendency of others may be to avoid the subject or to repress any inclination to mention the child, perhaps with the best of intentions. They may not want to upset the parents or bring back painful memories. However, in reality, the parents *are* upset and the painful memories are rarely far from the surface. And in all likelihood, the behavior of others would be perceived as more sensitive, and thus more helpful, if the parents had permission to openly acknowledge their child and her or his life that has come and gone, especially if this is what the parents prefer.

It is important to be aware that when parents are denied the opportunity to speak and/or to express their emotions, they may grow resentful and angry. Such feelings may exacerbate their grief. What is more, the parents ultimately may choose to separate from these others whom they perceive as uncaring and insensitive (Knapp, 1986). And this kind of choice, although necessary, also adds to the sense of loss already being experienced. Indeed, the death of a child may be a loss that leads to many other losses.

Most significant in this regard is the loss of one's story about life and what it is all about. However false our assumptions may be, we tend, for example as noted previously, to believe that life is orderly, that children are born, that parents die, that each new generation succeeds the previous one. We also may assume that there is justice in the world, that bad things only happen to bad people. We may have put our faith in a loving supreme being and trusted that we live in a benign universe, that all is right with the world. Whatever our beliefs, we generally find them greatly confused, if not shattered, when we experience the death of a child. Indeed, "When you have lost a child, all that is left is to try to understand what you can" (Jurgensen, 1999, p. 162) We thus may find the need to seek answers in entirely new places and seemingly strange ways.

For example, although death previously may have been a fearful subject, one studiously to be avoided, parents may now find themselves desperate to understand what happens after a person dies. It therefore may be useful to encourage exploration of death in many cultures as well as in the context of a variety of belief systems. What is important at this point is to support the questions rather than attempting to provide answers. Also important is the need to refrain from making judgments about the kinds of explorations in which bereaved parents may choose to engage.

A typical concern of bereaved parents is the knowledge that their child is OK. They also long for communication with their child, which they may seek from nontraditional sources. They may turn, for instance, to any one of a number of available books describing contacts made by a medium with children who have died. These books certainly may be comforting as the messages often conveyed by them are that children who have died are doing fine and that they want their parents to be well. According to one source, "Children on the other side often encourage their parents to move on with their lives, caution them not to be overprotective of surviving siblings or overly worshipful of them simply because they died" (Martin & Romanowski, 1994, pp. 11–12).

Reading such books or even going to a medium may appear inappropriate or unacceptable to an outsider, but grieving parents deserve whatever consolation they can find. What everyone would do well to remember is that such pursuits will not take away the grief or the need to mourn. They may, however, provide a well-deserved and much-needed respite—however brief—from all the pain.

Similarly, parents may feel that they are receiving communications on their own but may be afraid to share their experiences with others for fear of either being considered crazy or having their hopes dashed, or both. Songs that come on the radio or the license plates on other cars may seem to be conveying a message from a child who has died. Or there may be more direct contacts, either through dreams, visions, or the sense of a presence in terms of sound, sight, or smell. In my own experience, significant objects moved often enough that I began to pay attention. And nothing could have been more bizarre or less believable than the following events which occurred some months after my son died.

My husband and I had made one of our regular visits back to St. Louis from our new home in Texas, to which we had moved 10 days after my son's death. While we were gone, we had put our dog, Ashley, in a kennel, as was our habit. As was her habit whenever we brought her home from the kennel, Ashley headed immediately for her water bowl and drank until she was no longer thirsty. On this particular day, after Ashley had finished drinking and had walked away from her water bowl, which was next to the white tiled kitchen wall, my husband asked me to look at the wall and tell him if I saw anything. What I saw splashed in water on the wall was my son's full signature, exactly as he would have written it. This is also what my husband had seen but didn't tell me until I had seen it, too. We wanted to take a picture but knew it wouldn't show up. My husband's story was that my son was trying to let us know he was with us, even in Texas, because it had been so hard for us to leave St. Louis, which is where we had all lived together.

This may seem to be a totally inconceivable story and certainly I thought long and hard before deciding to tell it here. However, I am aware that when I share it with other bereaved parents they nod in agreement and then feel free to tell me about their unusual experiences. As they are validated and assured that they certainly are not going crazy—or that if they are, they are not alone—they feel a great sense of relief. This, in turn, often helps in the process of restorying reality in such a way that eventually life may once again seem to make some sense and their grief may be eased.

Indeed, the search for understanding and, ideally, resolution following the death of a child generally is a long and painful process. What is called for throughout is sensitivity to what is going on, as nearly every belief formerly held may be called into question. Activities previously enjoyed now may seem meaningless; going to work may become a pointless endeavor. Life may seem hollow, empty. And as the days and months stretch into years, others may grow impatient, not understanding why it is taking so long. Relationships may be reevaluated and changed, or perhaps ended. Indeed, one of the relationships most at risk following the death of a child is that between parents.

THE RELATIONSHIP
BETWEEN GRIEVING PARENTS

Two of the greatest challenges for bereaved parents include recognizing that each may grieve in a different manner and finding ways to support each other despite the differences (J. R. Bernstein, 1997; Lindbergh, 1998). For example, one spouse may wish to talk whereas the other may prefer silence. One may be unable to focus on anything; the other may prefer to bury him- or herself in work. One may cry incessantly; the other may not shed a tear. One may feel that his or her grief will continue for a lifetime; the other may achieve a feeling of resolution quite early on in the process. One may wish to talk about the child who died; for the other this may be too painful. On any given day, one may be "up" while the other is "down." Responses such as these are all perfectly normal, but problems arise when one parent or the other has a sense that there is one right way to grieve or when one feels judged negatively for behavior that is different from that of the other. In reality, each person must ascertain the way that is best for him or her while recognizing that there are as many "right ways" to grieve as there are people.

When the members of a couple find themselves grieving differently and having disparate inclinations, they also may feel frustrated that their needs are not being met by the one person on whom they thought they could depend. At the time at which support is most necessary, the other spouse simply may not be able to provide it, or at least not in the way desired. Thus, one parent must feel that he or she has permission to seek assistance elsewhere if it is not available at home. Extended family members, close friends, clergy persons, and counselors all may be viable alternatives when the stress on the marriage becomes too great and the limits of what is possible for the couple on their own are exceeded.

Indeed, perhaps the most supportive behavior on the part of one spouse toward the other may be respect for his or her inability to provide what is being sought and the choice to look elsewhere to have one's needs met. Similarly, it is important for spouses to avoid making assumptions about what the other is thinking, feeling or doing. Although often difficult, what is called for is communication that allows for the expression of each person's preferences, including the desire to be silent or to withdraw.

However, given the level of stress being experienced by both partners, effective communication may be difficult to achieve. Certainly it is not unusual for tempers to flare and for even the smallest issues to become the source of major conflict. What is more, each spouse may evidence moments of seemingly "irrational" behavior. What has become irrational, however, is life. When nothing makes sense any more, how can one be expected to behave rationally? Thus each spouse must learn patience, tolerance, and forgiveness if the couple is to survive the tragedy and remain together.

In addition to differences in mourning styles, there also may be variations between spouses in terms of their desire for reentry into the world. This includes the willingness, or not, to engage in sexual intimacy, to interact socially, to return to work, or to do anything just for fun. For one spouse, taking part in any of these activities may seem like a betrayal of the child who has died. Or, the choice to participate may be followed by feelings of guilt and thence a return to a period of withdrawal. Indeed, for those grieving, the process of recovery often may seem to involve taking one step forward and two steps backward.

Spouses also may find themselves in conflict around religious or spiritual beliefs and behaviors. One spouse may feel totally alienated from the spiritual realm, and the other may perceive it to be a great source of comfort. Or, one spouse may have newly created beliefs that the other finds distasteful. What is more, one member of a couple may feel that the other has gone off the deep end in terms of explorations in this area.

Another source of tension may arise around what to do with the dead child's room and/or how to handle his or her things. For some, it may be important to leave the room as it was. For others, giving everything away and getting on with life may seem the better option. Once again, learning to honor and respect differences and to seek a reasonable compromise is the key.

Finally, even though not justified, spouses also may blame each other for the death of the child. Our natural inclination is to want to find a cause, to point the finger at somebody. Unfortunately, in the context of grief and confusion, inappropriate blaming may occur, thus adding to the grief process for everyone. Indeed, this process may be so destructive that couples are advised to seek outside help at the first indication of its presence: "If help is not sought and the problem not resolved, all hope of a meaningful life is nearly gone for both the blamed and the blamer" (Schiff, 1977, p. 65).

From my own clinical experience and that of others (Shapiro, 1994) as well as according to research data (Nolen-Hoeksema & Larson, 1999), it would appear that there are two basic scenarios that tend to play out following the death of a child. On the one hand, there are those couples for whom the loss is more than the marriage can bear. Ultimately, the members of these couples choose to part from each other and to go their separate ways. However, it is worthy of note that "in the majority of cases in which bereaved parents divorce, the death is only the last straw in the demise of the marriage" (J. R. Bernstein, 1997, p. 104).

On the other hand, some couples find themselves drawn closer together as a function of having experienced the loss of a child. For them, separation is unthinkable in the context of the new bond that has been forged, one that holds them together more securely than ever before. As one mother reports after the loss of her daughter in an automobile accident:

> "Her death has brought us closer together. My husband is more compassionate and listens to me more. More in tune to my feelings than before" and "the pain and harshness of the type of death has strengthened the marriage. We've been able to communicate so much better than before. I've come to appreciate my son and my husband a lot more." (Lehman, Lang, Wortman, & Sorenson, 1989, pp. 355–356)

Whether parents find themselves drawn closer together or they choose to separate, they continue to be challenged in terms of how best to respond to their other children. Indeed, when a child dies the family is affected in many ways. The parents are grieving and so also are any surviving children. Just as spouses look to each other for support, children look to their parents to take away the hurt as well as to continue to love and care for them and to meet their needs much as they did in the past. But the parents may find it difficult to respond as they might have done previously.

RESPONDING TO THE OTHER CHILDREN

Although parenting, even under the best of circumstances, is perhaps one of life's most rewarding undertakings, it also can be one of its most demanding. The impact of parenthood on both the individual lives of the parents and the couple relationship in terms of such issues as energy drain and lack of privacy is well-documented (Barnhill & Longo, 1978; Carter & McGoldrick, 1980; Duvall, 1962). Indeed, caring for and providing for the well-being of children, supporting their educational and social needs, and maintaining a supportive and nurturing environment constitute a full-time commitment, one that requires tremendous emotional, as well as instrumental, resources. It is therefore not surprising that the ability to meet such demands and to parent effectively following the death of a child is often sorely compromised.

Bereaved parents generally find that they have little to give to their other children: "Parenthood now becomes walking and talking and listening and hearing someone else at a time when it takes everything just to think or function for oneself" (Schiff, 1977, p. 84). Parents may be so immersed in their own grief that they are unable to see either the needs of others or the impact of their behavior on those around them. Thus, in addition to the sadness they also are feeling, the other children may feel confused about where they stand, about their relative importance to the parents (Bouvard & Gladu, 1998). The surviving children therefore may withdraw from their parents or may engage in antisocial behavior. Or, at the other end of the spectrum, they may repress their own feelings and needs and attempt to take care of their parents, either directly through parent-like behavior or indirectly by attempting to become perfect, to avoid making waves or causing additional stress.

On the other hand, parents may be making what they feel are monumental efforts to respond well to their surviving children, only to learn at some later date that the messages sent were far different than the message received. In my own experience and that of many others (e.g., Schiff, 1977), the parents certainly were less effective than they perceived themselves to be in terms of providing comfort to their other children. However, as my very wise daughter noted many years later, by way of consolation, "You know, Mom, I noticed that they weren't handing out instruction booklets at the funeral."

That, of course, is part of the dilemma. Parents don't even know how to handle their own grief let alone that of their other children. Nor are they able to figure out how to be parents in a world that has gone topsy-turvy. What is more, the learning that comes from experience often arrives too late to help in the early, most vulnerable period of the grief process.

Thus it would behoove those who desire to help grieving parents to be aware, first of all, of the importance for the parents of maintaining a connection with their surviving children. To avoid the creation of either emotional or physical distance, parents might share what and how they are feeling rather than withdrawing and attempting to hide their sadness and tears. They might also do well to reassure their other children that they are still important and much loved. Certainly the parents may own their feelings of powerlessness regarding the death and yet also they must convey, somehow, that they are capable of handling life and all its challenges, including taking care of all their children.

Parents must make time to be with their surviving children, being sure that the surviving children don't feel ignored or that their feelings are somehow less important than their parents'. It also is essential that the parents maintain some semblance of order. Thus, for example, there continues to be a need for regular routines and rules as well as consequences for breaking them. As always, children derive a sense of security from knowing both that there are limits and that they will be enforced. Similarly, the generational boundaries need to be enforced and it is inappropriate for parents to look to or expect their children to take care of them.

As overwhelming and seemingly impossible as all this may sound, everyone is helped with their grief when there is both a recognition of what is at stake and a focus on creating a context that is nurturing and supportive despite the pain. Rather than doing irreparable damage, the family thus may not only survive but also may grow following the loss of a child. To accomplish this goal, however, it also is important to be aware that although the death of a child is challenging at every stage of development, there are some unique aspects worthy of consideration when the child dies either during pregnancy or in early infancy.

WHEN A BABY DIES

Although family members and friends often are at a loss as to how to help the parents of a child who has died, they generally are most in the dark when it comes to providing support following a miscarriage or early neonatal death. They would be quite unlikely to suggest to the parents of older offspring that such a loss is something the parents will get over in time, or that they are young and surely will be able to have another child, but all too often these are the responses when a miscarriage occurs or a baby dies. However, such messages can be extremely hurtful, often isolating the parents, who thus feel even more alone in their grief given the lack of understanding by others of what is happening for them. Indeed, the significance of this kind of loss and the grief it entails cannot be underestimated:

The loss of a baby is the loss of a person. All parents who are positive about their pregnancy include their baby not just in their plans for the future but in their present lives too, so that even before birth, a baby begins to be considered, loved and cared for. A baby's death is also the death of a person *who would have been*. It means the ending of dreams and hopes and plans, the loss of a future. Even a baby lost in the earliest stages of pregnancy may have this significance for the parents. Parents may also have invested so much of themselves in their baby that when the baby dies, a part of them dies too. Parents who lose their first baby lose their new identity as parents; those who already have children lose an expected new member of their family. (Kohner & Henley, 1997, p. 9)

Regardless of the circumstances, therefore, what seems crucial is to avoid minimizing the experience in any way. Beginning with medical personnel and continuing with other family members and friends, the bereaved parents need validation regarding the extent of their loss. They also need permission to express their feelings and to talk as much as any other parents who have lost a child. Mothers, in particular, need to have their physical as well as their emotional vulnerability recognized given all the hormonal changes they are likely to be experiencing. Both parents need a great deal of information as well as the answers to questions about which they may not even be aware they need to ask.

For example, depending on the age of the baby at the time of death, parents may need to know where she or he will be, how they can see him or her if desired, ways in which they may participate in the preparation of the baby's body, the opportunity to take pictures or have hand- and footprints, religious or other services available in the hospital, cause of death, and postmortem information. They also need to be advised regarding future possible pregnancies, available support services, appropriate follow-up care, and external resources should they need further assistance. All this is in addition to information that is needed about funeral and burial arrangements and options (Kohner & Henley, 1997).

Another important issue for parents who lose a baby concerns the decision, in the midst of mourning, regarding whether or not to become pregnant again. Many young parents choose to have another child, sometimes as a way of dealing with their grief. Many often subsequently deliver perfectly normal, healthy babies. The problem is that all the predictable worries of pregnancy are often multiplied many times over for parents who have previously lost a baby. Thus, the 9 months of waiting becomes a period of great fear and anxiety rather than one of excitement and anticipation. As one mother reported to me, "I was scared to death throughout the whole process—worrying about whether the baby would be normal. I freaked out if I didn't feel the baby kicking."

For the parents who do become pregnant again there also may be mixed emotions as happiness about the new baby triggers feelings of guilt related to the child who died. Some parents choose not to have another baby, believing that they just could not endure another experience of loss, potential or otherwise. And some parents who would like to have another baby find that they cannot, for a variety of reasons. In each of these cases, further loss and grief need to be recognized and accommodated, which requires sensitivity to the uniqueness of each situation and enough time to allow healing to occur. The good news is that healing is possible and that ultimately the changes that evolve following the death of a child, whether early in life or at any point thereafter, can be positive in spite of also being painful.

AFTER A CHILD DIES

Losing a child inevitably alters personal perspectives in many ways. When parents subsequently reflect on what has changed for them they find, for example, that life no longer seems quite as pure and wonderful as it once did (J. R. Bernstein, 1997). Gone is a sense of innocence or naiveté about reality. And even the happiest of occasions may have an undercurrent of sadness.

Parents who have lost a child also are likely to notice that their priorities have changed as they have sought to bring meaning and purpose back into their lives (J. R. Bernstein, 1997). How time is spent and who it is spent with become much more important in the awareness that life is both precious and fragile. Similarly, what is valued tends to shift, with more of a focus on relationships and the ability to be compassionate toward and supportive of others and less of a focus on the acquisition of material goods or personal status.

Whether the response of bereaved parents is to become more aggressive or more fatalistic relative to the process of attempting to control reality, these parents also recognize the way that life can spin out of control in an instant, and certainly without warning (Bernstein, 1997). They have a much greater awareness of their vulnerability and an understanding that despite their best intentions, they may not be able to protect their children. Lost is the sense of comfort and security that existed prior to the death of the child. Gained is a more realistic picture of the vicissitudes of life as it really occurs.

Death also acquires a whole new meaning following the loss of a child and there is much less fear of the unknown (J. R. Bernstein, 1997; Shapiro, 1974). Many bereaved parents expect once again to be with their child, which brings a positive dimension to the thought of their own dying. Indeed, some may look forward to death as a release from the excruciating pain they are experiencing. Some also experience an increased ability to be with others who are dying and/or to call on the deceased child to be there to help with the process. Bereaved parents have had an intimate acquaintance with death which may desensitize them in many ways.

Indeed, and perhaps most significant, parents who have moved through the trauma of having a child die often find that they feel a much greater sense of competency in terms of both emotional resources and practical abilities (J. R. Bernstein, 1997; Bouvard & Gladu, 1998). Having faced the most dreaded and worst possible experience imaginable, life thereafter loses much of what previously was perceived as threatening or frightening. Thus these parents may sense the following:

> If you have withstood the fall of an empire you are invincible. You know what you can survive. You are strong, you have needed your strength and you are proud of it. The only thing that could drag you under would be a completely different kind of fall. Which plucks you gently. So you fall gently and very far. So gently that you do not make a sound as you touch the bottom. No more sound than you would make if you were to pronounce the word disappearance. (Jurgensen, 1999, pp. 163–164)

THERAPEUTIC CONVERSATIONS
AND REFLECTIONS

∽

David was a happy, healthy 7-year-old, his father's namesake, and his mother's delight. He had a sister who was 2 years younger whom they all adored and life in his family was good. One afternoon, however, while playing with some friends in the yard in front of his house, he darted into the street in pursuit of a ball and was killed instantly when he was hit by an oncoming car. When his father arrived home from work shortly thereafter he was greeted by a scene which included his wife in hysterics as her son was being placed in an ambulance, a crowd of neighbors, one of whom was holding his

---

crying daughter, the driver of the car who was sitting on the sidewalk slumped over with his head in his hands, several police cars, and flashing lights everywhere.

As David's father recounted this tale, his grief and pain were still quite evident despite the fact that 2 years had passed since the accident. He spoke with intensity, through clenched teeth, all the while fighting to control his emotions. David's mother, on the other hand, cried freely and often had difficulty talking as she described the horror of the entire experience. What had brought them to therapy was a pattern of conflict followed by distancing and withdrawal that had been increasing in recent months.

Although initially they had been able to comfort each another following David's death, over time anger on the part of his father and feelings of guilt on the part of his mother had hampered their ability even to be respectful let alone supportive of one another. Dad had become more and more immersed in his work and Mom had become less and less effective in her ability to care for their home and daughter. Now Mom wanted to become pregnant again, to have another child, but Dad simply was not interested. Indeed, he was not even sure that he wanted to stay married.

For David's dad, the loss of his son, his first-born child, had shattered his world. For a time he had attempted to numb himself to the reality by drinking but soon realized that this was not going to help him or anyone else. So he had once again invested himself in his career. He had found himself coming home later and later, not wanting to deal with the situation at home, and particularly with his wife's constant crying and her incessant talk about David and what had happened.

David's mom felt rejected by her husband, which just added to her misery. In the immediate aftermath of her son's death, she had had a great deal of help from friends and neighbors and was able to talk and cry whenever she felt the need. However, as time went by and she was more and more on her own, she found herself unable to function. She had become extremely overprotective of her daughter, fearful that something might happen to her as well. And her husband's rejection only added to her misery.

As the couple shared more of their story, it became apparent that David's dad did indeed hold his wife responsible, at least on

(cont.)

some level, for his son's death. He felt that if his wife had been supervising the children more closely, David would not have run into the street and he would still be alive today. Despite the fact that the children often had played in the front yard and that David had been warned and knew about the dangers of their high-traffic area, he couldn't seem to get past his anger at his wife. And although she knew in her heart that she had not done anything unusual on the day of David's death, she had also been beating herself up for not having been more watchful.

To begin to help this couple, it seemed appropriate to go back to the beginning, to find out about the families in which they had grown up and to hear more about what had brought them together, what they had loved and appreciated about each other. As they described their early years together, their similar backgrounds and compatibility, their hopes and the fulfillment of the dreams that the birth of their two children had represented, they were able to remember that theirs once had been a very strong relationship. They recalled how blessed they had felt, which of course only exacerbated their feeling of loss when David died. However, once they recognized that underneath the current hostilities and sadness a firm foundation existed on which a new relationship might be built, we were able to begin to focus on healing.

Attendance at a support group for bereaved parents supplemented therapy and enabled this couple to learn more about their different styles of grieving as well as to find validation of their experience. In addition, as we worked together, David's mom and dad were able to learn how to talk together once again, to express their feelings and concerns and to request the behaviors each desired of the other. We also devoted a great deal of time to considering how they might make sense of their loss and honor the memory of the son they had so dearly loved. When the time seemed right, we created together a ritual of forgiveness of self and other with an emphasis on moving beyond past hurts and thinking about how to create a more satisfying future together. This was a long, slow, and often painful process, but in time David's parents were able to recommit to each other and to their family. They even began to think about the possibility of having another child. Fortunately, although it was close, they had not waited too long before seeking outside help.

CHAPTER 7

When a Sibling Dies

✌

I am the fifth of five children. In my family there were three girls, then a boy and then me—a girl. Throughout my childhood and early adolescence, I was partic- ularly interested in and aligned with my brother. I was often accused of being a tomboy because I preferred my brother's company and his activities to the "girl" interests of my sisters. My brother was 2 years older than I was and I idolized him. I looked up to him as knowing everything and being able to do everything.

When I was 13 years old and my brother was 15 years old, he was killed in an automobile accident. My life was forever altered.

Initially I was in total disbelief: He could not be badly hurt, he was strong and healthy. When I was told he had died, I met this news with a total lack of understanding and appreciation of what lay ahead.

My happy-go-lucky temperament left; I became very distressed and ex- tremely serious. My distress was worry about him and me: Where is he? Is he OK? What do I do now? My seriousness stemmed from the realization that if this could happen once, it could happen again: What or who would be next? My concern for the safety of others in my life continues to this day and has not less- ened much in the subsequent 33 years.

After my brother died my family members disengaged from one another. There was just too much pain and fear. Both my parents began to drink heavily, literally spending all day at the bars. My two oldest sisters, both of whom were married, put their energies into their own families and my other sister left for col- lege. It felt and looked to me as if I had lost everyone. I spent many days and nights alone, literally.

My self-imposed isolation was further facilitated by my friends' avoidance of any topics of my brother and/or his death: They did not talk about him, al- lude to experiences they had had with him, or acknowledge my history with him. At times I had difficulty remembering who of my friends actually had

125

known him. Looking back on this, I imagine that no one wanted to hurt me by talking about him. However, the net effect was that I had no one to talk to about this gaping hole in my life. I felt like a pariah with people circling around me—they connected by their innocence about death and me tarnished by my experience of it.

I did not demand attention. I wanted to fit in, to go back to the time when I was the same as my friends. So I colluded in the silence. Secretly then I began to question my own memories of my brother: What was he like? What interests and experiences had we shared? Further, I became increasingly alienated from my emotional self, as if I had not been impacted by this tragedy at all.

I began to focus on being totally independent and put my energy toward achievement in academics and athletics. Socially, I felt like an outcast. I did not want to get close to anyone for fear of losing him or her: I preferred counting on myself. I became very introverted and anxious. I was anxious about wanting to connect with others and dreadfully afraid to do so.

Finally, after years of a self-imposed, goal-directed orientation to my life, I sought counseling. It was then that I began to accept that, truly, to have loved and lost was preferable to having never loved at all. I decided to pursue relationships and human contact again. Eventually I was successful in this regard.

Today I am happily married. However, my decision not to have children remains a direct consequence of my experience of my brother's death. I cannot tolerate my fear of the loss of a child. Consequently I have not put myself in a position where that might happen to me.

My relationship with my parents and siblings has never recovered enough to discuss the impact of my brother's death on me or them. Our loss remains a cross for each individual to bear alone. However, I can see the distress, seriousness, and anxiety in each one of us as a result.

—TVF

Although the significance of the relationship between parents and children, as well as that between spouses, is a given in our society, the same generally cannot be said for the relationship between siblings. Indeed, although "sibling rivalry" is a common enough term and, in fact, often has been the focus of research, little attention has been given to the dynamics of the ties that bind sisters and brothers together, either as children or as adults. Therefore, when the relatively recent book *The Sibling Bond* (Bank & Kahn, 1982) was published, it was advertised as "the first major account of the powerful emotional connections among brothers and sisters throughout life." According to the authors of this book, the patterns of attachment between brothers and sisters are both extremely complex and quite unique. It is their position that there is a link between siblings that is pivotal in many ways, regardless of whether the relationship is friendly or hostile. They explain as follows:

> [T]he sibling bond is a connection between the selves, at both the intimate and the public levels, of two siblings; it is a "fitting" together of two peoples' identities. The bond is sometimes warm and positive, but it may also be negative. Thus, for example, rivalrous siblings who hate each other can be considered to be "bound" if their identities have any influence on one another. Through the sibling relationship, one gets the sense both of being a distinct individual and of constancy through knowing a sibling as a predictable person. Even when the relationship is uncomfortable, brothers and sisters derive a sense of a familiar presence, however upsetting. (Bank & Kahn, 1982, pp. 15–16)

In other words, the way in which a person with one or more siblings defines or sees her- or himself in the world is inextricably bound up with her or his interactions with the other child or children in the family. In addition, as others have suggested, a significant aspect of one's personal identity and orientation to life may arise as a function of one's birth order, or sibling position (Hoopes & Harper, 1987; Sulloway, 1996). Indeed, as noted many years ago (Toman, 1961), the behaviors and inclinations of, for example, the older brother of a younger sister may differ dramatically from those of a younger brother of an older sister.

At the same time, relationships between siblings are more likely than any other type of family alliance "to be characterized by ambivalence or conflict" (Nolen-Hoeksema & Larson, 1999, p. 45). Starting with competition early in childhood and continuing far into adulthood, brothers and sisters may resent and/or harbor negative feelings about one another. They may vie with each other for their parents' attention or just to equalize or surpass perceived differences. They may resent assumed inequities in their treatment by others. Unfortunately, regardless of the degree of closeness—whether they are forced by circumstances and/or choose to continue to be involved in each others' lives or whether they prefer silence and separation—the tensions and conflicts between sisters and brothers may remain unresolved. In the event that one of the siblings dies without a resolution of negative feelings and ill will, the surviving brother or sister is faced with the task of coming to terms with the situation on his or her own.

Conversely, siblings who have struggled with each other for years may finally reach a point of resolution only to lose each other when death snatches one of them away. In this case, sadness over the loss may be compounded by several other factors. There may be regret for not having repaired the relationship sooner. There may be guilt for things said and done as well as things left unsaid and undone. And there may be sorrow about what might have been in terms of the potential of the relationship in the future.

In the case of siblings whose relationship has always been solid, perhaps becoming even more valued through the years, the death of a special person may create an extremely deep void for the survivor. Lost is the companion of one's childhood, someone who shared all the vicissitudes and triumphs of growing up, someone with whom to compare notes regarding life in their family of origin. Lost also is a friend, a trusted person who could always be called on for help and whose acceptance could be counted on regardless of circumstances.

Thus, whether embattled or beloved, the bond that is severed by the death of one of the siblings is likely to constitute an event of major proportions. Added to this is the fact that demographic changes in our modern era have altered the context of the sibling relationship, thus heightening the significance of a loss in this area. On the one hand, there is no reason to expect that the relationship will end, but on the other hand, its existence has become somewhat more precious.

To explain, as noted in the previous chapter, the death of a child is much less likely to occur today than was the situation in earlier times. Accordingly, parents no longer feel a need to have large numbers of children in order to ensure that some will survive into adulthood (Aries, 1962). Further, many young people currently are waiting longer to get married and, even when they do, often choose to focus first on establishing their careers before having children. When they ultimately decide to start a family, they may only have time or the inclination to have one, or at most, two children.

For a variety of reasons, therefore, families, tend to be smaller today than previously was the case. Parents are likely to feel complete, as well as safe, with the arrival of their desired one or two children. Given these changed circumstances, not only is the death of a child a great shock to everyone involved, but for the brother or sister it may mean the loss of one's only sibling. The surviving sibling may suddenly find that he or she is an only child, one who has now become part of an "endangered species." And the only remaining partner for this sibling "in the dialectical dance for self-definition" (Bank & Kahn, 1982, p. 272) typically partici-pated in by brothers or sisters is the ghost of the dead sister or brother.

However, even in situations in which more than one child survives, there is still a huge gap, one that can never be filled. Indeed, the absence/ presence of the child who died is so strong that the sibling position held by him or her continues to exert its influence on the life of the family. Thus, for example, birth-order roles tend to remain consistent following the death of a child (Hoopes & Harper, 1987). In other words, even when a miscarriage occurs or a baby dies, subsequent children tend to take on the role consistent with the succeeding sibling position rather than that held by the child who died.

Thus, whatever the nature of the sibling relationship, and regardless of the time of life at which a brother or sister dies, sibling loss should not be dismissed out of hand nor should its meaning and impact be underesti-mated. Certainly there are instances in which so much distance has been allowed to develop that the death of a sibling is unlikely to cause much distress. However, it would be premature and inappropriate to assume that sisters and brothers will not be deeply affected by the death without first consulting the survivor and attempting to understand the relationship. And when the impact of the loss is one of significant proportions, those who desire to help would do well to become more sensitive to and knowl-edgeable about what it is that siblings may be experiencing. For those seeking to help long after the loss, a careful assessment of the experience also would be appropriate, perhaps even despite reluctance on the part of the survivor.

In this chapter, therefore, our discussions revolve around the follow-ing four areas. I begin with a look at the ways in which sibling loss may be overlooked, either by others or by the sibling her- or himself. Also consid-ered as part of this discussion are the ramifications of such behaviors (i.e., being overlooked and/or minimizing the experience oneself) for the brothers and sisters of a child who has died. I then move to an examina-tion of the impact of the parents' grief both on the surviving children and on the life of the family as a whole from the perspective of the siblings. The dimensions and consequences of the grief experienced by these sib-lings is the focus of the third section. Finally, I conclude with a consider-ation of various ways in which sisters and brothers may be affected over the long term by the loss of a sibling at various points in life. Throughout these discussions, the implicit emphasis is on ways in which children, teenagers, and adults may be supported in such a manner that their grief is respected and additional, unnecessary pain is avoided when a sibling dies.

THE OVERLOOKED LOSS

Given the relative lack of attention that has been directed to the relationship between sisters and brothers in general, it is little wonder that the grief experienced by siblings tends to be an area that is often neglected and truly misunderstood. Indeed, not only is this the case at a personal level, but until recently, sibling loss has been almost entirely overlooked in the literature on bereavement (Rando, 1988). And this situation exists despite the fact that some research has revealed that such a loss is comparable to that experienced by adults who have lost either a spouse or a parent (Nolen-Hoeksema & Larson, 1999).

Therefore, in the anguish and confusion that follows the death of a child, his or her siblings may find themselves being thrust into territory that is not only treacherous but also uncharted, without guides or even the most basic of supports. Indeed, an extremely crucial part of the dilemma siblings may experience following the death of a brother or sister is the lack of acknowledgment of or comprehension about either their situation or the dimensions of their grief. For example, concerned relatives and friends may ask surviving children how their parents are doing and completely forget to ask the same question relative to the siblings' well-being. Or, they may not speak at all to the surviving children about what has happened, offering their concern instead to others. Whatever their age or situation, siblings and their feelings tend to be either discounted or relegated to a secondary position:

> Losing a sibling is particularly difficult because the other people in our family are considered the primary mourners. When we lose a brother or sister as a child, all the attention is focused on our parents and we feel invisible in our sadness. When we lose a sibling as an adult, the sympathy is offered to the spouse and children of our sibling. Our own loss is very wrenching, and yet there may be no acknowledgment of it. (Bouvard & Gladu, 1998, p. 104)

In addition, parents may look to their surviving adult children to make decisions and handle various necessary duties without recognizing how distraught the siblings are. While sisters and brothers are also deep in grief and perhaps feeling overwhelmed, they may be the ones called on to handle relatives and friends who are besieging the family with phone calls and visits. And parents may seek emotional support from their surviving children, talking about their own pain and soliciting solace in ways that are inappropriate for these offspring who also are bereaved.

If the surviving children are young, parents may be so preoccupied with other important decisions that they fail to take time to actually check in with the children and see how they are doing. For example, they must decide what and how much to tell them about their sibling and his or her dying, whether or not to include them in the funeral process, and what to say about death in general. Indeed, they may be doing everything they think they can and still inadvertently may overlook the grief their surviving children are likely to be experiencing.

The siblings themselves also may overlook or attempt to ignore their own grief as they do very little sharing, either with their parents or with others. As adults, they may believe that what is expected of them is the ability to carry on and to deal with the loss on their own. As adolescents, a typical response is to withdraw, both from family and from friends, rejecting any attempts on the part of others to reach out to them and letting no one know what they may be feeling (McGoldrick & Walsh, 1991). Indeed, the experience may be just too painful to talk about and they simply may be unwilling to bare their emotions in front of others. And as children they also may fear doing anything to further upset their parents. In the words of a woman whose sister died when she was a young girl: "I knew that no one could touch me or meet my eye, or my sadness would come rushing out with such force I would crack into thousands of splinters. I could not crack, no matter what. I had to be everything for them. I had to be good" (J. Bernstein, 2000, p. 63).

What is more, siblings at any age may find that permission does not exist to address any aspect of the fact that a sister or brother has died. They thus find themselves acting in accordance with the family rules, however implicit, which require denial of what has happened and the repression of associated feelings: "Many children learn from their wounded parents that to raise up a dead sibling's image is treacherous or disloyal. Bereavement must remain a private matter; one must stifle or choke back sadness, anger, or happy remembrances. Entombed within this conspiracy of silence, the family tries to regain its balance, and life goes on 'normally,' in the pretense that the death has never occurred" (Bank & Kahn, 1982, p. 275).

However, to be ignored, to have one's emotions denied or neglected, or to have unrealistic expectations about what one is capable of handling on one's own is distressing under any circumstances. Such scenarios become even more difficult to deal with when one's world is in the process of coming apart. As discussed in Chapter 6, there is no question that the life of the family is thoroughly disrupted when a child dies. For everyone involved, everything is suddenly turned upside down. For the siblings as well as the parents, the lens through which life is viewed often changes dramatically. And the reality now perceived generally bears little resemblance to the one in which they previously existed. Most significant in all of this for the siblings of a child who has died is the transformation of their parents, which literally takes place before their eyes.

SIBLING PERSPECTIVES ON PARENTS

As noted in the previous chapter, when parents lose a son or daughter, they tend to find it extremely difficult to continue to respond effectively to the needs of their surviving children. They may be unavailable or they may have unrealistic expectations of these children. And even when they make an attempt to be supportive, to maintain some semblance of normality, their efforts often fall short of the mark. Indeed, all the former predictability and stability of family life tend to be completely destroyed in the presence of grief for the child who has died. The siblings of this child, therefore, are faced with a variety of losses, losses unique to them and their situation.

Not only have they have lost their brother or sister, but they also have lost the reassurance derived from the assumed ability of their parents to handle whatever life has to offer. Lost are their former perceptions, however naive, of the people on whom they previously were most able to count. And they are likely also to be in the process of losing their sense of security as their parents start behaving in new and perhaps strange ways. In addition to being inconsistent, their parents now may appear extremely vulnerable. They may refuse to speak to the surviving children about their dead brother or sister, or they may idolize him or her. They may become overprotective or they may withdraw. In all likelihood they simply are unable to do a good job of helping the other children deal with the grief that they also are experiencing. It is not surprising, therefore, that whether the outcome is either positive or negative, the relationships between the siblings of a child who has died and their parents are likely to be forever changed.

For example, it is not unusual for siblings to feel emotionally abandoned, to experience themselves as being alone and unloved in the days, months, and even years following the death of a brother or sister (J. R. Bernstein, 1997; Schiff, 1977). In part, this perception may evolve from resentment about not being allowed time alone with their parents because of all the other people who suddenly are flooding their home. In part, it also may be triggered by frustration with unsatisfactory explanations given by parents about the cause of the death (Bouvard & Gladu, 1998).

As they grow older and more aware, siblings also may feel anger about many of the decisions their parents made at the time of the death, perhaps about excluding them in various ways because they were too young. For those allowed to attend and participate in funerals, there may be anger about the whole process, seeing it not only as intrusive but also as too costly, too long, or simply lacking in meaning. Teenage children also may resent parental expectations regarding participation in family rituals. Particularly distressing for them may be the requirement that they go to the cemetery. In the words of one young woman who had not visited her sister's grave since her death:

> "Sometimes, I think about going but I never do, and if I did, it would be by myself. Not with my parents. I resent their insistence that I go. Their loss is not my loss. By the same token, my loss is not theirs. If and when I visit my sister's grave it will be by myself. It will be a very individual and personal thing for me. I'll be there someday. Not yet, though. And certainly not because my parents badger me about it." (Schiff, 1977, p. 90)

When reflecting back on the experience, many siblings report that they felt more than abandoned, that they felt almost rejected by their parents. Their perception is that their parents expended insufficient effort on their behalf. It is not surprising, therefore, that a common reaction, particularly for teenagers, is to try to spend as much time as possible away from home. Encouraging this tendency is the desire to escape from the pervasive feeling of sadness and the presence of death which they associate with life in their own family. This situation is further exacerbated when parents become angry at their children for not wanting to stay at home but fail to try to understand the reasons for their children's choice to stay away.

Siblings also describe feelings of both anger and abandonment as a function of the loss of consistent discipline and the lack of a requirement to obey rules that once characterized their family. Suddenly, where they are and what they are doing doesn't seem to matter very much. All that seems to be important is that they, too, don't die. Thus, one surviving sibling remembers of her parents: "[T]hey fell into a deep sleep as soon as I came home at night. They had not noticed that I had dyed my hair black the week before, or that, when I paused at their door to say good night, I was sometimes so drunk that I could barely stand. That I was alive was enough" (J. Bernstein, 2000, p. 12).

At the same time, however, those who have lost a sister or brother also may be receiving messages from their parents, either directly or indirectly, that life is inherently dangerous and something to be feared (Bank & Kahn, 1982). Despite the absence of rules and structure, therefore, surviving siblings initially may find themselves becoming overly cautious. Subsequently, they may have to struggle, often in an extremely risky manner, to prove to themselves, and perhaps to others, that they will not suffer the same fate as their brother or sister who has died.

In addition, siblings may feel that they are being treated inappropriately as they are expected by their parents to become more like their dead sister or brother and/or to be a source of comfort to their parents. In the context of such expectations they not only become angry but also may perceive that somehow they are no longer important to their parents, or as important as their dead sibling. And this, in turn, may lead to resentment of the child who died and further grief over the loss of the family that once was. Indeed, for some, there is a sense that their parents were never able to come to terms with the death of a brother or sister in such a way that the family was able to regain a sense of coherence and normality.

Finally, siblings may fear becoming a burden, one that their parents are not able to bear. They may come to the conclusion that their parents are too vulnerable to be able to handle them or their needs. In response, the surviving children may choose to react with hostility or they may attempt to become perfect, or both. Whatever the choice, however, their own burdens are increased by the perceived absence of appropriate parental support.

The context of sibling loss is thus one characterized not only by much pain but also by an absence of acknowledgment and support as well as the presence of chaos and confusion. Added to this are the unique reactions each child has to the death of a brother or sister as a function of the type or cause of death, the life stages of those involved, and the nature of the relationship between the siblings. Indeed, sibling grief is a complex process containing many dimensions worthy of further attention.

SIBLING GRIEF

When focusing on sibling grief, most important of all is the recognition that surviving siblings are likely to be struggling with a variety of reactions, not only to their parents and others in their world but also in terms of their own shock and disbelief. In the first place, they simply may not be able to comprehend what has happened; they may be unable to believe that a brother or sister has really died. For a young child there literally may be no way to explain or understand that death means that her or his sibling is gone forever. For the older child, belief in one's invincibility and sense of immortality may preclude, at least temporarily, acceptance of the death of a sister or brother. And for adult siblings, particularly those geographically separated, "There is no acute absence to signal to you that he or she is permanently gone" (Rando, 1988, p. 157).

When siblings do eventually come to grips with the reality of the loss, they may find that they now feel much more vulnerable than previously was the case. Children often feel a sense of lost innocence (J. R. Bernstein, 1997) as they recognize that people of their own age can indeed die. Those old enough to consider some of the broader ramifications may become aware of shared genetic factors predisposing them to similar illnesses if a particular medical condition was the cause of death (Rando, 1988). And all siblings also suddenly may feel that they have aged 10 years in 10 minutes as they are forced to bear the heavy burden of their grief and acknowledge as well the fact that their family is shrinking.

In addition, as siblings begin to deal with the actuality of the death they are quite likely to experience a wide range of emotions, including "guilt (for survival, health, past actions, or jealousy), sadness, hurt feelings, loneliness, anger, confusion, fear, difficulty sharing feelings, disbelief, apathy, and numbness" (Nader, 1997a, p. 19). In fact, the list of possible reactions is probably endless. However, though all these responses may be normal and predictable, they are nevertheless challenging. And perhaps most difficult to deal with are the feelings of guilt which are likely to emerge and which may take many forms.

For example, survival guilt may be experienced as the brother or sister of the deceased child begins to feel that a mistake was made, that it was he or she who should have died. Such feelings may be evoked without a rational cause but may be exacerbated when the sibling sees the degree to which his or her parents are inconsolable and becomes increasingly aware of the inability of his or her presence to alleviate the pain the parents may be exhibiting. The sibling thus sees him- or herself as somehow less important, which increases the guilt he or she may be feeling for being healthy and for having survived (J. R. Bernstein, 1997).

Younger children also may feel guilty for things they did or said to their sibling, perhaps even fearing that they somehow participated in or caused their sister's or brother's death. If the child who died had been ill for some time, they also may feel guilty for resenting their parents' lack of attention while their sibling was still alive. Indeed, they may feel guilty for whatever emotions are assailing them, for example, believing that it is wrong to be angry or upset.

Nor are adult siblings exempt from the emotional roller coaster. In this case, they may have feelings of guilt which have evolved as a function of such issues as ambivalence in the relationship with the sibling, relief at not being the one who died, and/or recent interactions which were less than ideal (Rando, 1988). Old tensions and resentments also tend to reemerge following the death of a sister or brother and their lack of resolution may add to the feelings of guilt on the part of surviving siblings.

Those experiencing such feelings are likely to be confused and further upset by them. For, at the same time, it is likely that they also are overwhelmed by great sorrow as well as sensations of loneliness and longing for the sibling who has died. Thus, whether they respond either by becoming numb and refusing to speak about what is happening or by attempting to find an outlet enabling the expression of feelings, they may be caught in a tangled web of emotions. And what others see on the outside may be different from what they actually are experiencing on the inside.

For example, in the effort to fill the void created by the child who died, a sibling may attempt to offer comfort and to meet her parents' needs by becoming perfect. And she may be silently abetted in this attempt by parents who fail to recognize what is going on. In the process, however, the sibling not only is denying her own reality but, of course, also is setting herself up for failure. In the words of the same young woman quoted previously whose main focus in life after her sister's death shifted to the attempt to be everything for her parents: "In this dreadful silent house, where no mention of my sister was made and no one cried, I tried my hardest to be good, because I was all that was left. But at every waking moment I knew that no matter what I did, I could never be good enough" (J. Bernstein, 2000, p. 66).

On the other hand, there are certainly some siblings who choose to reject such a role. What is more, they may become angry at being told that they need to live up to the memory of a dead brother or sister. They therefore may work hard at becoming totally dissimilar and respond by acting out in a variety of ways. Indeed, they may feel that they have to go to great extremes in order to be recognized as unique individuals rather than as replacements for the sibling who has died. The following story illustrates such a scenario: "Craig could think of only one way to escape an impossible rivalry with a dead brother. He would not compete. He would be as different as possible. The similarity between them created comparison, and in that comparison the living child paled before the memory of the dead" (Schiff, 1977, p. 92).

Given the nature of the burden created by the death of a brother or sister, it is therefore not surprising that the appearance of a variety of physical symptoms, often for prolonged periods, is quite common (J. R. Bernstein, 1997). In fact, some individuals are able to express their grief only through physical reactions. However, most people who are bereaved are likely to have some experience of bodily symptoms as part of the grief process (Rando, 1988).

Young children who have lost a brother or sister because of a physical illness are particularly susceptible in this area. If the death was caused by cancer, for example, siblings may "show signs of physical illness including complaints that mimic the symptoms of their deceased sibling" (J. R. Bernstein, 1997, p. 143). Other problems they may evidence include bedwetting as well as a variety of aches and pains throughout their bodies.

With older children, reactions to the stress of the situation may emerge in the form of various physical problems, some of which may even be a mystery to physicians. Sometimes the symptoms may fluctuate and change over time. In either case, it may take time and much support to sort out exactly what is happening. To illustrate, a young woman whose brother died when she was 20 years old recalls that during the following 2 years she experienced repeated episodes of difficulty swallowing, followed by fears about being able to breathe, which often grew into full-blown panic attacks. Her fears could be triggered by almost anything but she was particularly susceptible to instances she witnessed of labored breathing, for example, on TV or in the movies.

Over time, the young woman was able to recognize that her fears, in general, grew out of the experience of her brother's death and the sudden awareness of just how fragile life can be. Suddenly she was subject to numerous questions and concerns she had not previously considered. If life could end so abruptly as it did for her brother, why couldn't the same thing also happen to her? Having seen death at close hand, she no longer could take either her health or her life for granted. It now seemed to her that death could come at any time and without warning. Her particular fears about not being able to breathe, she realized, were connected to having seen and heard her brother following his placement on a respirator during the final hours of his life. It was only after she was able to make these connections that she was able to overcome the problem. Indeed, as with any traumatic experience (Figley, Bride, & Mazza, 1997), the aftershocks of sibling loss may continue to reverberate for many years following the actual death.

LONG-TERM EFFECTS OF SIBLING LOSS

The degree to which siblings manifest various emotional and physical reactions, as well as their subsequent ability to resolve the loss, is affected by a number of factors. The nature of the relationship that existed between the child who died and his or her brother or sister is extremely important in this regard. For example, if the ambivalence or hostility was great there may be either great guilt or great indifference. A sense of closeness and deep affection, on the other hand, may mean a loss of great magnitude for the sibling. However, in the latter case the pain may be diminished, or at least not magnified, given the good feelings about the relationship.

Also important to consider is the cause of death. As discussed in Chapters 3 and 4, anticipated versus unanticipated deaths are accompanied by many different issues and concerns. This is true not only for adults but also for children. Thus it is important to know whether the sibling's death was caused by illness, accident, or violence. If the survivor was a child, was she or he exposed to circumstances that were unusually cruel or harsh? How was the situation handled and explained? And at any age, was this the survivor's first experience with death?

Another significant consideration is the point in the individual and family life cycles at which the death occurs and the way in which appropriate developmental tasks and issues subsequently are supported, or not. If the family is able to acknowledge appropriately the form that grief may take for each individual, family members will have entry to a path toward recovery. If they also have avenues of expression and support, they can begin to walk this path. And if family members recognize and accommodate all the normal needs of individuals and families as they live, evolve, and grow through time, the healing process for all certainly will be facilitated (Shapiro, 1994). Thus, for example, it is important to be aware that despite fears about children's safety which may have been exacerbated by the death of a child, adolescence brings increasing needs for freedom. At the same time, although rules relevant when the children are younger need to be relaxed as the children grow older, adolescents still need guidelines, expectations, and consequences for inappropriate behavior. As young people are dealt with effectively, they receive an implicit message about the strength and ability of their parents, one that enables them to feel more secure both about themselves and about their family, despite their grief.

Closely related is the fact that how the loss is dealt with over time by other family members has an impact on the healing siblings are able to achieve. As young people learn through observation of others, and particularly their parents, that one can be happy as well as sad, that it is OK to laugh in spite of the pain, that life continues even when a life ends, they will be encouraged in their attempts to make peace with the death of a brother or sister. Conversely, when the grief goes underground, when nothing ever seems to be resolved, young people may see their families as having been destroyed by the death, or at least as existing in a dark place, forever after.

Indeed, the degree to which both communication (Baker, 1997) and the restructuring of family rules and roles are able to be facilitated will play a crucial role in the support of sibling grief. It is important to allow for the expression of feelings in ways that are appropriate for each person. Parents do not have to try to hide their grief from their young children; their children know that they are sad and this knowledge is less damaging than the pretense that everything is all right.

Adolescents typically withdraw, even under the best of circumstances. Thus they may need extra encouragement and permission to give voice to what is going on inside: "I could not speak of my own accord. I needed someone to shake the truth out of me, to slap me, to demand I tell the story, to use any means to make me speak her [sister's] name" (J. Bernstein, 2000, p. 116). At the same time, parents also need to remember that whatever they do, it may not be enough, that there may be little they can do to take away the pain of the loss: "I remembered, too, that nothing my parents did made me feel better after Laura's murder. When they tiptoed, it was the worst; when their voices were soft, it was the worst; then they said nothing and asked for nothing, it was the worst; when they wanted something, it was the worst. I had no comfort, no place to hide, no solutions for their problems, no salve for their wounds" (Bernstein, 2000, p. 170).

What parents can do is to be sensitive to and to acknowledge the turmoil being experienced by their surviving children. What others may do is offer support in this effort. Indeed, making recourse to assistance from outside the family from those who are not so overcome by grief may be highly appropriate and helpful.

Adult siblings, too, need recognition that they are primary mourners. It is interesting to note in this regard that along with the death of parents, sibling loss is most likely to profoundly influence and precipitate changes in perception about oneself, one's career choices, and one's priorities in life (Nolen-Hoeksema & Larson, 1999). And the siblings, themselves, also need to acknowledge how deeply affected they are and have been by the loss of a brother or sister. They need to take time to grieve, perhaps even demanding it when it is not forthcoming from others (Rando, 1988), and they need to find ways to express their pain.

As with the death of any loved one, many good things also may evolve from the experience of the death of a sibling. Perhaps because the survivors feel so ignored and have to struggle so hard to have their stories heard, they learn much that stands them in good stead as they go through life. However, when a sibling dies it behooves us to remember that these surviving brothers and sisters are generally the ones who will live longest with the loss. If life proceeds in the future in a somewhat more orderly fashion, that is, it is likely they will outlive their parents. And at the point of their parents' death they may find themselves to be not only the oldest living generation in the family but also alone in this position, with no sibling on whom to lean.

THERAPEUTIC CONVERSATIONS
AND REFLECTIONS

∾

Ellen and Susan were not only sisters, they were also best friends. They had had the normal squabbles as young children, but no matter how much anger they might display in the heat of an argument, by the end of each day their parents generally would find them sleeping together in one or the other of the twin beds in the room they shared. Ellen was 5 years older than Susan and her delight at the arrival of her baby sister had never diminished. Susan had responded in an equally loving way to her proud and protective older sister.

When Susan was 10 years old, she was diagnosed with CLL—a particularly virulent form of leukemia. She spent several years in and out of the hospital, enduring the various toxic treatments and all their attendant side effects. In time, to the great but guarded relief of her family, the cancer went into remission. Throughout this period her distraught parents cared for her, spent endless hours with her at the hospital and in doctors' offices, and helped her in every way they knew how. And for them, although she certainly did her share of complaining, Susan maintained as brave a facade as could be expected of any child her age.

It was to Ellen that Susan felt she could speak more freely of her anxieties, her fears about the future, and her frustrations as she grew older and experienced lack of understanding from peers and teachers. The girls, already close, became inseparable and during the early years of treatment, whenever Susan was well enough, Ellen included her in activities with her friends. After Susan's cancer went into remission, they were almost euphoric. They enjoyed shopping sprees together and going to see the plays that were Ellen's passion. They laughed and cried together and they schemed to play practical jokes on their parents. They also began to make a series of videos.

Periodically they would interview each other and talk about what was going on in their lives at that point in time. They also enacted some of the silly scenes of everyday life that had caught their fancy and just generally clowned around. When a tape was completed, they would then host a "showing." They would send invitations to close friends and family members, asking them to dress for the occasion and to come at the appointed time, and would serve refreshments as they enjoyed the video together.

After high school, Ellen chose to live at home and to commute to a local college while completing her studies. Upon graduation, she took a job in her hometown and moved to a small apartment not far from where her parents lived. Susan followed in her older sister's footsteps, attending the same college, but decided to live on campus. Although the sisters were not able to spend as much time together, they often talked on the phone and the visits they had became even more meaningful. They also continued to make their videos and host showings, which by now had become a family tradition.

In the middle of Susan's sophomore year, when she was 20 years old, the event everyone had feared but no one ever mentioned—at least publicly—occurred. Susan had a recurrence of her cancer. What is more, the prognosis was not very good. However, her par-

(cont.)

ents attempted to remain optimistic and denied what was happening long after it became clear that Susan was dying. Susan also continued to be brave and to express hope, especially in front of her parents. And once again, it was Ellen with whom she was able to be totally honest.

There was much that Susan wanted to say to her parents both about her life and about her death. However, she also wanted to spare them further anguish and she knew how painful it was for them to speak with her about the inevitable. So she and Ellen decided to make a final video. They continued to include lots of humor, but they also created a format that enabled Susan to speak about the various memorable moments in her life, to thank her parents for all they had done for her, and to offer loving messages to the people who had been particularly important in her life.

During this process Ellen and Susan, as usual, laughed and cried together, often pointing the camera at themselves as they sat with their arms around each other in Susan's bed, which now occupied an honored spot in the family room of their parents' home. Susan also gave Ellen instructions on the final showing, which was to occur the night before her funeral in place of a viewing or wake. Just before she died, Susan told her parents what she and Ellen had done and let them know of her wishes in this regard. Everything else she left to them to decide.

I know what a great loss Susan's death was for her parents as well as for her sister, but I also am in awe of the strength and the support the two young women were able to provide not only for each other but for those around them. Susan's parents have the gift of an incredible visual record of their daughter as she was in life and as she prepared to die. In addition to this living monument, her sister also has the memories of a loving relationship and the knowledge that she and Susan made the most of the time they shared together. None of this will fill the void, but it certainly will help with the grief they all undoubtedly will experience for the rest of their lives.

CHAPTER 8

When a Parent Dies

◞

The phone call telling me that my mother had cancer came just before Christmas, 22 years ago. To this day I am sorry that we did not just cancel our Christmas plans, pack up the kids and presents, and scrape the money together to fly back home. However, no one knew much about the diagnosis or prognosis, and Mom put up a confident front so that we wouldn't worry too much.

In early January, my brother called to let me know that Mom was hospitalized because of jaundice, that the physicians were now sure that the liver was affected and that a liver coma might occur at any moment. It was during the blizzard of 1978, when the East coast was blanketed with snow and ice and a state of emergency kept most vehicles off the road. To me, this was a dire emergency. I booked a flight for the next day and my husband drove 5 hours through horrendous conditions to get me to the airport. I was so distressed that I aroused suspicion when I gave my maiden name to the agent at the gate—something I had not done since the first weeks of my marriage 10 years earlier.

Coming back to my childhood home with my mother in the hospital was an eerie experience. My father and two older brothers had waited for me with anticipation. While I am the youngest in the family and had been "babied" quite a bit growing up, I now suddenly and without conscious intent was cast into the role of my mom's successor—guarding and nurturing everyone's physical and emotional needs. I was keenly aware at that first meal around our dining room table that my father wanted me to sit to his right, the place usually reserved for my mother. The symbolism of this invitation was not lost on me. My father did not like my refusal.

The role change from youngest in the family to "female in charge" who would know how to set things right, much as my mother always had, was amazing. My father and brothers looked up to me and left many decisions, particularly those pertaining to my mother's care and the running of the household, up to me. These were completely new dynamics. In retrospect, I realize that be-coming the caretaker of my mother and father saved me from my own grief and despair at losing the mother I loved.

A gall bladder bypass operation gave Mom some relief but also confirmed the diagnosis: advanced pancreatic cancer. "What is it?" my mother begged to know, but was then seemingly satisfied with vague replies. My father refused to believe the diagnosis and got angry at my brothers and me whenever we would mention it or talk about my mother's impending death. On the one hand, he ac-cused us of wanting our mother dead and on the other he could be heard sobbing uncontrollably during the night only to tell me, "it's okay, go to sleep," through the closed door.

Most hours of each day I spent at my mother's bedside. My brothers had gone back to their families and my father kept up a minimal work schedule. Mom and I had many conversations, revisiting events in her life, some of them difficult—like her relationship with my grandparents, her in-laws; some of them sad—like the loss of her younger brother in World War II; and some of them happy—like her relationship with a close friend whom she had met as an adoles-cent.

Mom asked a few times what the doctors were telling us outside her door but then turned away without wanting to hear the answer. The morning when I decided that I would tell her the diagnosis, on the way to the hospital I suffered an anxiety attack for the first time in my life. Later, Mom listened calmly to what I told her. Her eyes filled with tears and then she said, "I am not afraid to die. God forgives my mistakes."

Everyday my father would sit by my mother's bed and squeeze her hand so hard that she flinched. He could not tolerate the bed railing up because it seemed to separate him from Mom, so he put it down as soon as he entered her room in spite of mom's feeble request to keep it up. Initially, I spoke up for Mom, ex-plaining that she felt protected by the railing and that her skin had become so sensitive that Dad's squeezes hurt. Predictably, as I can see now, Dad became annoyed at my interference. It slowly dawned on me that my parents were act-ing out the last chapter of a 40-year marriage and that I had no right to inter-vene. It was not my place to try to change their marital dynamics.

Mom came home to die, and we kept a vigil for the last two nights, taking turns sitting with her, holding her hand, reading Bible verses to her or singing her favorite hymns. Mom fell into a coma that lasted 36 hours. I remember clearly her belabored breath, her moaning and writhing with pain, her suddenly clear words before slipping back into the dusk. The night she died I was holding Mom's hand and beginning to speak to her softly, saying, "I don't know for sure what is coming afterward, but I trust that you will be safe and well and happy.

You can let go, we love you so much." As I relaxed my own breathing, Mom's breath got calmer. An hour before my brother was to take over the vigil, my 5-year-old son began to cry upstairs. I tried to take my hand out from Mom's to check on him, but Mom held tight. When I whispered to her, "I have to briefly check on your grandson, he is crying," she immediately let go of my hand—in spite of not having reacted to anything we had spoken to her during the 24 hours prior!

Mom died right when my brother took over the watch. My father must have sensed it and seemed to appear out of nowhere in the room. It felt like a holy moment, as if Mom's soul or spirit were still present. For quite a while after her last exhalation we all stood by her bed. It was as if an invisible presence was in the room that kept us spellbound and in awe. I can only describe it as being touched by the holy, by eternity, by grace and unbounding love.

It was just past midnight when we called the nurse, who came right over to help me wash and dress my mother and comb her hair. It was a very moving, loving, sacred time—except for the scare I got when we lifted Mom's back and head and the last air escaped her mouth, 2 hours after she had died!

The morning of the funeral my children were busy in their bedroom. As we left, my daughter, age 6, showed me three pictures she had made for her grandma: a flower, a star, and a butterfly. My son clutched the pictures which he had produced under his sister's tutelage: a heart and a candle. I was amazed to realize that this was all my daughter's doing. At the funeral the children suddenly let go of my hand, tiptoed to the open coffin, and lay their presents next to Mom's hands. Everyone's eyes teared up.

It is amazing how quickly I transferred all my care and attention from my mother to my father—again postponing my own grief. My father was so absorbed in his despair that all my "doing" was a welcome means to going on.

Two separate incidents brought me to deal with my own sadness and loss. About 2 weeks after the funeral, back at home, I stood in the aisle of a grocery store, looked at a can of tomatoes and burst out crying. I cried so hard that I had to abandon my shopping and drive home bleary-eyed. My mother had loved tomatoes—and I had loved my mother.

The second incident took place a few days later. I sat at my son's bedside to say good night, and he looked up at me with all the innocence and inquisitiveness of a 5-year-old and asked, "Mom, is grandma now turning into a skeleton?" I could only say, "Yes, and it is so sad," and call my husband to take over so that I could cry.

From that point on I began to punctuate my stories with phrases such as, "When Mom was still alive," or "After Mom's death." Her death became a definitive marker for me. And I changed a lot through it all. Mainly, I lost my in-

nocence and carefree ways. I also, without conscious decision, changed my
wardrobe. About 8 years after my Mom's death my husband noted, "I think
you are coming out of mourning—you are adding some color to your beige and
black wardrobe!" He was right!

—IH

For good or ill, parents have an influence on the lives and development of
their children that is unsurpassed by and more long-lasting than that of
any other relationship. Those who assume the roles and responsibilities of
parents become the primary attachment figures for their offspring, consti-
tuting their whole world during the period of infancy. It is from parents
that children first learn about such basic issues as nurturance and security.
And with every interaction they are inculcated with the values, beliefs,
thoughts, feelings, indeed the very framework according to which their
parents live their lives.

All of us look to our parents to guide and protect us as long as we are
in their care, and sometimes far beyond that point. Throughout our for-
mative years our parents are crucial to the process of identity formation
and the creation of perceptions we have about ourselves as well as others.
As adults, whether we choose to emulate or reject what we have learned
from them—either by what they did and said or by what they didn't do or
say—the behaviors as well as the voices of our parents, and thus their influence, go with us. Therefore, the death of a parent, whether biological
or adoptive, is likely always to be a significant event and an important
milestone.

At the same time, however, there is perhaps no other loss with
greater diversity of meaning for survivors depending on factors such as
age, individual development, gender, and family life-cycle stage. That
is, for a young child the loss of a parent is both unthinkable and life-
changing, whereas for a mature, older adult it is highly predictable and often assumed to be less disturbing. Similarly, the ability to understand the
meaning of the death of a parent varies considerably as a function of one's
level of cognitive and emotional maturation. What is more, the death of a
mother tends to have a different impact than does the death of a father,
and this impact may differ for sons as opposed to daughters. And when
the last parent dies and orphanhood becomes one's reality, it, too, has
widely varying ramifications depending on the ages and developmental
stages of the surviving children.

Also influencing the course of bereavement following the death of a parent is the fact that just as relationships between parents and children tend to be among the most powerful and important, they also are likely to be some of the most complex and stressful. Conflict and controversy are as normal a part of the ebb and flow of relationship patterns between parents and children as are love and laughter. Indeed, much of the growth of children evolves out of the struggle to differentiate themselves and to become individuals who are connected to yet distinct from their parents. This process of individuation often continues long into adulthood. Throughout, feelings may vacillate tremendously and children ultimately always may think of their parents with mixed emotions. For example, in the words of Oscar Wilde, "Children begin by loving their parents; after a time they judge them; rarely, if ever, do they forgive them" (*Oxford Dictionary of Quotations*, 1980, p. 753). Thus, the particular circumstances characterizing the relationship at various points in time are sure to wield their influence on the grief experienced by a child when a parent dies.

Accordingly, all children who lose a parent are affected not only by the death but also by various issues surrounding the loss. Along with the characteristics of those involved as well as prior patterns of interaction, this also includes both the manner of the death as well as the availability of support. Indeed, in the relationship realm, young children are not as likely to have been engaged in struggles that seriously tested the nature of their connection with their parents. Rather, the three major concerns they tend to have following the death of a parent include the following: "(a) Did I cause the death to happen?; (b) Is it going to happen to me?; and (c) Who is going to take care of me?" (Nolen-Hoeksema & Larson, 1999, p. 122). Of crucial importance for children in this age group, therefore, are issues of survival and concerns for the self.

By contrast, relationship issues tend to rise to the fore for children in their teen years. It is a well-known fact that the period of adolescence is often quite turbulent as young people seek greater autonomy and parents learn how to adjust the balance between control and freedom. The loss of a parent at this point in the family life cycle may be complicated by much internal conflict on the part of the surviving young person. There may be guilt and self-blame about having desired to be rid of parental authority. There may be hostile feelings toward the parent, a product of the ongoing battle for independence. And there may be a lack of validation for such feelings on the part of others whose perceptions of the deceased parent are far more positive (McGoldrick & Walsh, 1991).

Still other issues may emerge for the young adult whose parent dies. Just when the child is likely to be investing energy in the establishment of a separate life (e.g., in college, in a career, in new relationship commitments), the pull back into the family of origin that is likely to follow the death of a parent may seem to threaten her or his newly defined sense of self. Thus there may be a perceived need to create even greater distance and to underestimate the importance of relationships with siblings, the surviving parent, and other relatives. Or, conversely, a decision to return to the family fold may impede normal development for the young adult who takes on caregiving duties and then chooses to remain in this role for an overly prolonged period (McGoldrick & Walsh, 1991).

Recently married or young couples with or without children may similarly be torn between feelings of responsibility for their old and new families. For them, however, a focus on obligations toward the family of origin may slow the process of creating and adapting to their newly formed marital/couple system. Added to the strain this may put on the relationship between the couple may be a sense of urgency or pressure to begin having children. On the other hand, the presence of a spouse or partner, as well as of children, in the life of the adult child may diminish the sense of desolation often experienced when a parent dies (McGoldrick & Walsh, 1991).

These are just a few of the many stresses and strains that may affect the grief process following parental loss. To further understand the variety of contexts of grief following the death of a parent, this chapter considers several topics in greater depth. First I will examine the impact of the death of a parent on young children. As the area of bereavement most often studied and most frequently discussed, there is much we can learn not only about how children respond to the loss of a parent but also about how best to help them with their grief. Next, I focus on adults, considering the way bereavement is affected by age as well as the way the loss of a parent may affect sibling relationships. The third area of concern is that of orphanhood, or what happens when the last parent dies, both for young children and for adults. In the fourth section I address gender issues. Accordingly, I compare the differing ramifications for females and males when they lose either a mother or a father. Finally, this chapter looks at family structure and the influence on the grief process of various changes which may be necessitated by or may emerge following the death of a parent. As we shall see, an incredibly broad range of potential issues and reactions may be evidenced by children when one or both of their parents die.

PARENTAL LOSS IN CHILDHOOD

Just as it is important to be aware that the bereavement process varies across the entire lifespan, it is equally crucial that we be sensitive both to the unique ways in which children in different developmental stages tend to experience the death of a parent and to the distinctive manner in which they generally express their grief (Steinberg, 1997). Perhaps most significant, however, is the need for recognition that "children *do* grieve" (Rando, 1991, p. 199). What is more, they are likely to need help in the process of coming to terms with this grief.

The possible symptoms children may evidence following the death of a parent are many and varied. Such a list includes anger, anxiety, behavior disturbances, cognitive difficulties, denial, depression, developmental delays, eating problems, fears that the surviving parent also will die, feelings of abandonment, guilt, hopelessness, insomnia, loss of trust, phobic reactions, regression, and restlessness (Rosen, 1986). Though they thus quite typically experience as full a range of emotions as those who are older, the key to the degree to which childhood bereavement is successfully negotiated seems to lie with "the way the surviving parent responds, the availability of social support, subsequent life circumstances, and continuity in the child's daily life" (Nolen-Hoeksema & Larson, 1999, p. 111).

The responses of an infant to the lapses in the nurturing process that are likely to occur following the death of a parent usually are discomfort and tears, both of which may be relieved rather quickly when these gaps are filled (Rando, 1991). By contrast, slightly older children may display a sense of distress which continues over a longer period. They may repeatedly request that the lost parent return and may reject anyone who attempts to act as a substitute for their missing mother or father (Raphael, 1983). For them there is little understanding that the loss is permanent.

Children between the ages of 2 and 5, however, may be assisted to understand the meaning of death (Raphael, 1983). Although they thus can be dealt with in an honest and direct manner they also may revert to behaviors of an earlier age (e.g., bedwetting). At the same time, trying to protect them by avoiding discussion of the death in their presence or excluding them from funeral activities and services is likely to increase rather than alleviate their anxiety (Rando, 1991). Similarly, it may be harmful should adults in their world fail to recognize the children's grief, which in this age group is likely to be demonstrated on an intermittent rather than a constant basis.

Between the ages of 5 and 8, children may experience a sense of guilt about their parent's death or they may act as if the death has not happened or is not permanent (Rando, 1991; Raphael, 1983). Given the greater ability of children at this age to understand the meaning of the loss, coupled with a lack of coping skills, they may revert to denial in order to contain their emotions or avoid the appearance of being considered babyish should they show their grief. Although they therefore may attempt to hide their tears, they are likely to be helped most by encouragement to openly acknowledge and express their feelings (Nolen-Hoeksema & Larson, 1999).

The reactions of children between the ages of 8 and 12 tend to mimic or be similar to those of adults. Children at this age are able to comprehend the nature of death in all its finality and universality. They thus are likely to experience an increase in their fears about both their own mortality and that of their surviving parent (Raphael, 1983). Anger in the form of increased irritability and defiant behavior is a typical reaction and needs to be understood for the grief response that it well may be.

As mentioned previously, adolescence generally is synonymous with much turmoil and instability. Young persons in this age group are experiencing monumental changes at many levels—biologically, emotionally, cognitively, and socially. Their struggle at this point is first and foremost to achieve a sense of personal identity and self-understanding, a daunting challenge all by itself. Add to this mix the death of a parent and the result is a recipe for confusion, fear, and concern not only about how they will fare but also about how they will be perceived by others. What is more, adolescents tend to believe that their experience is unique to them and that others are not capable of understanding the grief they are feeling (Nolen-Hoeksema & Larson, 1999). Thus they may be overwhelmed by a variety of intense emotions and their grief is likely to be expressed in intermittent, brief outbursts (Raphael, 1983).

Knowing the typical responses of children of various ages to the death of a parent may enable those who would help to have a greater understanding of their behavior. Indeed, as we are able to see through the various facades to the underlying pain, we may be able to support rather than attempt to inhibit normal grief responses and encourage the expression of feelings in a healthy manner. As part of this effort, it is essential that adults communicate with children honestly and directly, using language that is understandable relative to the developmental level of the survivors. What is more, children need to receive information about a parent's death as soon as possible after it occurs. Ideally, it should be provided by the surviving parent in a safe environment. The explanation should be truthful and should remain consistent over time. As part of this conversation, children should be given reassurance regarding the continuation of love and care. They also should receive validation for their feelings as well as recognition of the fact that all family members will be going through a process of sadness and grief which each person will be expressing in her or his own unique way (Rando, 1991).

In addition, it is important that children be given the opportunity to participate in the various rituals and activities related to both the funeral and the mourning process. "Although there is clinical evidence to suggest that children who are excluded without choice may become very angry, there is no evidence that allowing a child to attend a funeral is harmful" (Nolen-Hoeksema & Larson, 1999, p. 132). If the child chooses not to participate, however, she or he should not be forced to do so. If, on the other hand, the child chooses to participate, she or he should receive clear explanations regarding what to expect (Rando, 1991) and accommodation should be made for the fact that the child may lose interest and want to leave a particular function early.

Continuing opportunities to take part in rituals that commemorate the parent who has died also may be helpful to the grief process. Further, as part of the ongoing effort to help children come to terms with parental loss, they may be encouraged to create inner constructions or representations of the deceased parent. Such constructions may help to maintain a sense of connection with this parent (Nickman, Silverman, & Normand, 1998). Surviving parents may play a significant role in their creation process in several ways. They may encourage the expression of memories and feelings. They may support a realistic assessment of both the negative and the positive qualities of the parent who died. And they may allow children to describe their feelings about what they have lost or miss most. Further questions which may aid the creation of a viable construction of the deceased person, for both the surviving parent and the child, include the following: "Do you ever talk to him?" "Does she answer you?" "Do you dream of him?" "Where do you think she is now, or do you not think of her as being in a particular place?" "Do you sense him near you? Is that a good feeling, or not so good" "Are there things you'd like to be able to tell her?" (Nickman et al., 1998, p. 133).

At the same time, regardless of the strategies chosen to help them resolve their grief, children must be allowed to remain children. They must be understood and supported in age-appropriate ways. And their needs must be provided for despite the burden now being carried by the remaining parent. Thus, it may be extremely important to search for and enlist the support of extended family members and friends to help with the process of regaining balance and maintaining some sense of stability through the transition. Understandably, this is likely to present a huge challenge, for as the child loses a parent, the remaining parent loses a spouse. Indeed, the impact of the loss of a spouse will be discussed in great detail in Chapter 9. For now, however, it is time to turn our attention to an examination of the experience of the death of a parent when one is an adult.

PARENTAL LOSS IN ADULTHOOD

Perhaps the most surprising aspects of the death of a parent are the nature of the grief and the degree of sadness experienced by surviving adult children. Certainly we all know and expect that someday our parents will die. In fact, as adults the death of a parent is one of life's most predictable events and, according to many, does not pose the same kind of challenge as do other kinds of losses. For example, we are told the following:

> In today's society, in the cycle of human development, it is normal and natural to lose your parents when you yourself are an adult. The death of parents is the single most common form of bereavement for adults. Depending on their ages and on yours, death is usually more or less expected. In contrast to the death of a child, it is consistent with the laws of nature. In contrast to the death of a spouse, it usually does not deprive us of our primary sources of companionship and identity. And in contrast to the loss of a brother or sister, it is usually less threatening to us personally. (Rando, 1991, p. 137)

Nevertheless, no matter how predictable or expected, for many adults the loss of a parent may be followed by an extended period of anguish and bereavement. And this period may be more difficult as a function of the grief and turmoil whose profoundness was unanticipated. Thus, for some, the death of a parent does the following:

> [It] shakes up the very foundations of our lives. Daily routines are disrupted, assumptions about life and death jolted, values challenged. The gut-wrenching awareness of our own mortality, of the fragility of life, of the depth and intensity of our feelings, of the power of love and the reality of our aloneness thrusts us into a relentless and often painful questioning that probes to the depths of things, searching for meaning. (Kennedy, 1991, p. 56)

Once again, however, it is necessary to make a distinction, this time between the reactions of young adults as compared to those of older adults, to the loss of a parent. For the former group, issues around separation still may be looming large. Guilt about negative interactions therefore may be more a part of the grief response. In addition, young adults may experience a sense of frustration that resolution of conflicts with the deceased parent now is not possible. By contrast, it is likely that older adults have achieved a greater sense of acceptance and mutual understanding in the relationship with their parents. Indeed, the loss may be even more poignant given the recognition of their parent's unconditional love and support despite difficulties they may have experienced through the years (Bouvard & Gladu, 1998).

What is more, young adults usually are more dependent on their parents as their primary source of emotional support. They also are not likely to have many others in their world who can understand what they are experiencing. Thus, although they may feel a sense of release from parental surveillance, they also may feel abandoned and uncertain about how to make their way from this point onward. Similar contradictory and paradoxical reactions include both exhilaration and terror (Kennedy, 1991). For older adults who have lived longer and been through more, the death of a parent is not as unique an experience. They have friends and family members who have been through the same kind of loss and are therefore likely to find more support for their grief. At the same time, however, the death of a parent may bring to an end what was a close and intimate relationship. Further, given the presence of their own children, it also may mean the loss of a grandparent who played an important role in the life of their own family of procreation.

The younger adult, who is just beginning to create an independent life, also is challenged with the resurgence of grief as each succeeding milestone is achieved without the presence of the parent who has died. Significant events such as graduations, weddings, the birth of a child, career successes, holidays, and birthdays thus become bittersweet experiences, with happiness tinged always by a longing for the missing parent. On the other hand, although older adults may have friends and family members who are more understanding of their grief, they may be faced with colleagues at work or in other similar contexts who are unable to acknowledge or accept the depth of their emotions. Indeed, given the relative lack of value placed on the elderly, the loss of an aged parent generally is not given great significance in our society (Bouvard & Gladu, 1998).

Finally, the relationships between siblings also may be affected differently by the loss of a parent at different stages of development. When a young adult loses a parent, it is quite possible that one of the oldest surviving children may choose to take over the role of that parent. This may engender hostility and resentment on the part of younger siblings if not handled appropriately. Dissension and conflict also may emerge if and when the surviving parent decides to remarry and the siblings disagree in their reactions. On the other hand, for older adults who are more likely to have drifted apart in the process of establishing their own lives and families, the death of a parent may mean the loss of the person responsible for unifying the family or at least bringing various members together from time to time. And at any age older adults may harbor feelings of either resentment or gratitude relative to the way the parent was treated or cared for by siblings prior to her or his death. Similarly, how responsibility for the surviving parent is to be handled may bring sisters and brothers closer together or drive them apart.

As may be apparent from this discussion, parents continue to play a significant role throughout the lives of their children. Although children may respond differently as a function of their particular life circumstances at different points in time, the grief felt at the death of a parent is likely to be intense and should not be ignored. As younger adults we may attempt to push it aside and move on with life. Nevertheless, it exists and is likely to surface from time to time. As older adults we may be able to achieve a greater level of acceptance. However, there also may be both a pervasive sense of loss as well as the need to repeatedly remind oneself that the parent is no longer here. What is more, when both parents are gone, regardless of our age, we may find that we have moved into a whole new realm of experience.

WHEN THE LAST PARENT DIES

The idea of orphanhood for a young child conjures up all kinds of negative images and related concerns. Both real-life stories and those found in fictional literature provide many examples of poorly treated children, separated siblings, and a life that is forever diminished following the death of both parents. Fortunately, in this day and age, the likelihood of children being abandoned as a function of the death of both parents or the absence of other caregivers is relatively rare and thus basic survival issues are no longer of primary concern. Rather, assuming continuity of care, grief reactions following the loss of the second parent are likely to be similar to those following the loss of the first parent. As children grow and are able to understand this loss in its fullest sense, however, they also may find themselves facing some additional difficult issues.

Today, there is much greater awareness of the impact that the loss of both parents has on adults. Indeed, we now are much more likely to recognize that becoming a member of the oldest surviving generation is a life-altering event, albeit one that happens later in life. Given the increase in life expectancy, we can anticipate the presence of and a relationship with parents long into our adult lives. At the same time, the loss of both parents is a milestone that 75% of the adult population is likely to have passed by the time they have reached the age of 62 (Brooks, 1999).

Many factors enter into the bereavement process when we become "orphans," no matter at what age or the age at which we become aware of the broader ramifications. For example, with the death of the last parent we must accept the reality that we are no longer somebody's child (Brooks, 1999). And given the unique bonds between parents and children, when we have lost both of our parents we generally have lost the most likely source of unconditional love and concern that anyone will ever feel for us (Rando, 1991). No longer can we look to the people from whom we might most reasonably have expected to receive support and validation. Also lost are the people for whom we often found we were trying to prove ourselves as well as the opportunity to continue to do so.

In addition, when we have lost both of our parents the primary connection we had with our past also is obliterated (Brooks, 1999; Rando, 1991). As the repository of shared memories and family stories, parents tend to provide the link to past generations, to our childhood, and to many of the subsequent events leading to the present. Thus offspring may find themselves feeling intensely alone, despite the presence of a spouse, children, or other family members. And such feelings of aloneness may be particularly acute if one is an only child or there are no other surviving siblings.

What is more, parents tend to provide a cushion between life and the reality of death. With their demise we are likely to confront more directly our own mortality. And this awareness may be emphasized as we find ourselves having to take over many of the responsibilities for the family (Rando, 1991). Thus we may feel our age more and have an increased sensitivity to the fragility of life. At the same time, though we may mourn the ability to look to our parents for advice and guidance we also may experience a feeling of liberation at our newly acquired sense of autonomy and freedom (Brooks, 1999).

Several relationship issues also may come into play in the bereavement process following the death of the last parent (Brooks, 1999). We may find that our grief over the loss of our first parent is either reactivated or allowed to emerge fully for the first time when the last parent dies. For example, we may have been very young when the first parent died. Or, we may have been so involved with the care of the surviving parent that our attention was diverted and we did not allow ourselves to grieve fully. Moreover, having had the additional time with the last parent and the opportunity to form a closer relationship in the absence of the first parent, we may find the grief experience following the death of the last parent to be even more intense.

Finally, sibling relationships may become even more significant than was the case following the death of the first parent. In addition to the issues previously discussed, siblings now also may be faced with decisions regarding funeral arrangements as well as the division of their parents' worldly goods. In either case, this may be a source of tension and conflict. Certainly stories abound regarding the severing of family ties that resulted from disagreements over who is to inherit what, particularly when the parents did not specify their wishes or did so only in a general way.

Further, without parents to pull them together, siblings may no longer feel an urge to maintain their relationships. Indeed, much of the semblance of relationships between siblings may have existed only to satisfy the parents' need and desire for closeness between their offspring. Without this impetus, there may be little left to hold them together. What is more, with the loss of a family home at which to gather, there no longer may be sufficient reason or energy for siblings to attempt to get together. On the other hand, and perhaps more unusual, siblings who previously had drifted apart may feel motivated following the death of the last parent to reconnect in order to maintain or regain the feeling of family. Thus, following the death of the last parent, "Some sisters and brothers draw closer together, but others drift apart and experience two crushing losses at once, the death of the parent and the end of family life" (Bouvard & Gladu, 1998, p. 193).

Becoming an orphan therefore may be understood as an experience of great significance, one that is likely to affect all surviving children regardless of their age. They must learn to live in the context of new circumstances requiring the creation of a new relationship with the world and others in it. As part of this process, survivors must redefine themselves as people without parents to whom they may relate as children or from whom they may continue to expect, perhaps unrealistically, their desired responses (Rando, 1991). As always and as this chapter particularly emphasizes, how the bereavement process proceeds will depend on the various factors unique to each situation. For children who have lost one or both parents, certainly one such factor worthy of further consideration is gender.

GENDER ISSUES

Whether the parent who died was the mother or the father and whether that parent is survived by a daughter or a son may influence the way that surviving children respond to each other and to the world as well as to the death of both the first and the second parent. For example, in general, daughters who have lost a parent may feel more depressed than sons as a function of the fact that they tend to remain more closely tied to their parents than do sons, even as adults (Nolen-Hoeksema & Larson, 1999). At the same time, the meaning of the loss, for sons as well as for daughters, changes depending on the gender of the parent who died.

Mothers typically provide the very foundation on which we build our lives. They are the archetypal source of comfort and care, the ones who, at least in theory, love and understand us better than all others. As we grow and change, we may go through difficult periods, but nevertheless, we retain the idea of mother as someone who will always be there for us. What is more, for an adult daughter, the loss of a mother may mean the loss of a friend and companion. An adult son, who may not have been as closely attached, still may feel great grief at the death of a mother because, of the two parents, she was the one with whom he was able to be more open and expressive (Bouvard & Gladu, 1998). Thus, we may need to recognize that "when you lose a mother, the intervals between grief responses lengthen over time, but the longing never disappears. It always hovers at the edge of your awareness, prepared to surface at any time, in any place in least expected ways" (Edelman, 1994).

Moreover, just as the loss of a mother seems to have a greater impact on females than on males, it also may be particularly significant when the death occurs early in the life of the daughter:

Unlike the adult, who experiences parent loss with a relatively intact personality, a girl who loses her mother during childhood or adolescence co-opts the loss into her emerging personality, where it then becomes a defining characteristic of her identity. From learning at an early age that close rela-

> tionships can be impermanent, security ephemeral, and *family* capable of be-
> ing redefined, the motherless daughter develops an adult insight while still a
> child but has only juvenile resources to help her cope. (Edelman, 1994,
> p. xxv)

Indeed, the aftermath of the death of their mother, for both young girls
and boys, may be a sense of arrested development. As several of my clients
have expressed, at times they feel that they are reacting as though they
continued to be the age they were at the time of their mother's death.

And when the parent who died was a father, what then is the impact
on sons and daughters? More to the point, perhaps, we may ask and seek
answers to a most important question:

> Who were our fathers? They were heroes. They were villains. They were in-
> dulgent, withholding, stern, or sentimental. They were affectionate. They
> were aloof. They were men striving to live up to the ideal of a society that
> put great demands on them. They were responsible for the economic sur-
> vival of their families. Some caved in under the pressure, forever affecting
> the lives of their children. More were constant and loving providers, sources
> of great strength for their families. (Brooks, 1999, p. 129)

It is typical for both men and women to measure their sense of personal success against the standard set by their fathers. They thus either attempt to attain the level achieved by their fathers or compensate for
whatever it was they perceive their fathers did not achieve. In addition, it
is to fathers that we often turn for advice and guidance about such matters
as finances and careers and it is their sanction we often seek for our life
choices. Sons, in particular, tend to look for their fathers' approval as they
strive to equal or better their father's performance in the professional
realm. And sons are the ones who may feel abandoned should the loss of a
father occur early in the process of establishing a professional identity
(Bouvard & Gladu, 1998).

When a father dies, it is the eldest son who typically is expected to
assume the role of head of the family. However, this responsibility falls
largely in the financial realm, while daughters are expected to take on the
nurturing role. Thus, it often is assumed that daughters will look after the
surviving mother when the father dies. And when it is the mother who
dies, daughters often are expected to become caretakers not only of the
surviving father but also of other children and extended family members.
Such added responsibilities tend to increase the distress experienced par-

ticularly by daughters. (McGoldrick & Walsh, 1991) and also may exacerbate tensions between siblings.

The response of younger boys and girls to the death of a parent also may vary. Boys may begin to engage in such antisocial behavior as drug use, fighting, stealing, or withdrawal. Girls, on the other hand, may act out sexually and seek through relationships with friends the means to overcome their loss. And for both groups, the death of a parent in childhood may affect their ability as adults to form and maintain intimate relationships. Marital difficulties may ensue when the parent who died and the child were of the opposite sex. By contrast, parenting problems may be more likely when the parent who died and the child were of the same sex (McGoldrick & Walsh, 1991).

Thus in many ways gender is a crucial variable in the grief process. As with all the factors that may come into play, however, the degree of their impact is a function of the way the person who is bereaved is responded to and the ability of the family to adapt and reorganize itself. Indeed, the structural changes that inevitably occur may have the greatest influence on the child following the death of a parent.

FAMILY REORGANIZATION
AND STRUCTURAL CHANGE

A story I have heard repeatedly in the context of therapy details the experience of both young and older children in the aftermath of a parent's death. That is, the surviving parent who is left with a broken heart, sometimes little or no parenting experience, and perhaps several children often turns to drugs, alcohol, or other men or women to assuage the pain. Then, before coming to terms with the loss of her or his spouse, this surviving parent remarries with the hope of replacing the lost parent and thereby solving the family's problems. The stepparent, who may or may not be equipped to handle the situation, nevertheless finds him- or herself in an already difficult spot that is compounded by the grief reactions of everyone involved. It is not surprising, therefore, that in later years what clients find themselves experiencing, perhaps as much as or more than the loss of their parent, is the loss of the family that occurred when the parent died:

> [Indeed] researchers have found that children who lose a parent need two conditions to continue to thrive: a stable surviving parent or other caregiver

to meet their emotional needs and the opportunity to release their feelings. Sheer physical care isn't enough. The child who can express her sadness and who feels secure in her environment is the one most likely to integrate the loss and avoid serious ongoing distress. But the child who faces continuing difficulties—a father who can't stop grieving, a stepmother who rejects her, an unstable home life—can end up a long way from the point where she once began. (Edelman, 1994, p. 8)

Awesome responsibilities are thus placed on the surviving parent at a time when dealing with them probably could not be more challenging. What is more, even when such responsibilities are handled well and even when the children are older, the choice of the surviving parent to find another meaningful and committed relationship may be met with hostility and resistance. That is, the children may feel threatened when their sole parent begins to date. And they may reject their parent's new spouse should she or he ultimately decide to remarry. The children may feel that the surviving parent is attempting to replace the parent who died. They may fear the prospect of an outsider coming in and changing their family. Or, they simply may want to hold on to the idea of the family as it used to be.

However, change is the rule following the death of a family member. And when a parent dies, the reorganization that is required may be monumental. Helping the surviving parent understand the grief and the resistance to change that his or her children are likely to be experiencing may facilitate both the grief process and the ability of the family to create and adapt to new roles. And such assistance also requires understanding that the surviving parent also becomes a bereaved spouse when a parent dies.

THERAPEUTIC CONVERSATIONS AND REFLECTIONS

Carolyn's story is long, complex, and sad. At age 30 she had been in and out of therapy for years, had been hospitalized several times, and had been unable to find a meaningful career. She was intelligent and had a great deal of potential that she invariably undermined by inappropriate attempts to change the situations in which she worked.

During the first 6 years of her life, Carolyn had been the late and much doted on fourth of her parents' children. When she was born, her older sister was 17 and her two brothers were ages 15 and 13. She had been spoiled by all her family members and basked in the glow of their love and affection. Things changed dramatically, however, when her mother died in a plane accident as she returned home from a visit with friends.

During the next 6 years of her life, until she was 12, Carolyn lived with her father. Her older sister was already married when her mother died, the older of her two brothers had moved away, and her other brother was in college. She saw them all periodically but was pretty much on her own during this period. Her father hired a housekeeper to cook and clean but did little to attend to anything but her physical needs. He never remarried and he became more and more depressed, eventually losing his business. Although Carolyn tried hard to cheer up her father, he had lost his interest in life. When she was 12, he died following a massive stroke.

After her father's death, Carolyn's siblings agreed that she would go to live with her sister and her sister's husband, who had three children younger than Carolyn. Carolyn had to move and change schools. She also went from being the youngest to being the oldest child and she had to adapt to a whole new family situation that was less than ideal for her. Her brother-in-law, who had agreed to taking her, seemed to resent her presence and was unprepared for the adolescent rebelliousness that emerged whenever Carolyn couldn't get her own way.

Her sister tried hard to understand and to provide a sense of security for Carolyn, but she, too, often became frustrated with the situation. She also was concerned for the well-being of her own children and was angry at the turmoil created by her younger sister's presence in the household. It was during this period that Carolyn began experimenting with drugs, alcohol, and sex. It was also during this period that Carolyn began to see a therapist, the first of many.

Carolyn graduated from both high school and college in the middle of her class. She had repeated episodes throughout of drinking too much and of being suspended for breaking rules. Hospitalized for the first time at the age of 16, her pattern with therapists, as well as with teachers and instructors, was to appeal to them as a needy child in the hope that they would respond to her as parent

(cont.)

substitutes. Often this worked for a time, but eventually Carolyn felt rejected as they began to set limits and attempted to establish more appropriate boundaries in their relationships. It was then that she would resort to threats of suicide.

Over the years, Carolyn held and left a succession of jobs. By the time she came to see me she also had been under the care of a variety of psychiatrists and had taken many medications, none of which had been particularly successful in alleviating her symptoms (she had been diagnosed with both anxiety and depression). Carolyn also soon revealed a pattern of minor physical ailments and frequent visits to physicians specializing in many different areas. She had a trust fund, established for her by her father, that had been her source of income since she turned 21, and that enabled her to live comfortably. Nevertheless, she was anxious to create a more meaningful life for herself.

I cannot claim that therapy with Carolyn was a great success. However, we took some small steps that it is hoped will enable her to create a more satisfactory lifestyle now that she has moved away. By establishing boundaries from the outset and refusing to respond as had others in her life, she learned that expressions of caring could take many forms. She often grew angry and frustrated with me, but I believe that as I held firm, for example, refusing to answer repeated phone calls, she learned to look to herself rather than to others to take care of her needs. In addition, rather than continuing only to lament her parents' deaths, she also came to appreciate how much both had given her while they were alive.

I said at the outset that Carolyn's story was long, complex, and sad. My sadness is mainly about what might have been for this bright and talented woman. I wonder how things might have been different if Carolyn's father had been able to find the support he needed to care for himself as well as for the emotional needs of his daughter. I wonder how Carolyn's sister might have been assisted with the process of including her in her family. I wonder how Carolyn might have been encouraged differently, in ways that allowed her most positive attributes to emerge. Most important, I wonder how she might one day learn to use all her experiences as a catalyst for growth and healing.

CHAPTER 9

When a Spouse Dies

❧

She was my student for 2 years in the high school where I was employed as a counselor. Special, but "one of my kids." After she went off to college, she came back for our homecoming. After a brief courtship, we married.

Three children later, a home with four bedrooms became necessary. In hindsight, I should have known something was amiss when I was still ferrying possessions from the "old house" to our "new house" at 4 in the morning on the day we had to be out. This was mid-February. Summer passed and fall came and still she had little energy.

When, over Christmas break, I was home for more than a day or two at a time, it finally occurred to me that a 27-year-old woman probably should not have to have a nap to be able to make it through the day. I requested that she visit our internist. She went with a girlfriend, then went shopping. Before she arrived home, the physician had called to refer her to a surgeon because of the results of her blood tests. She contacted the surgeon and was immediately scheduled for surgery.

The surgeon came to me before she was in recovery to tell me that he/we had a problem. Every pre-op test had suggested a bile duct blockage. Remove the gall bladder and clear the duct, and all will be well. He had found the duct clear but the liver appeared questionable. Didn't look like cancer, but it was only functioning at 5%–10%. Referral first to a gastroenterologist and then a hematologist whom I called for an appointment. I detailed all the relevant information to the nurse and was given a date a month hence. Two hours later the nurse called back saying the doctor wanted us to come in the next week an hour before the office opened. Suspecting she might be admitted to the hospital, we packed her bag.

She was admitted, and we were told she was also put "on the list." List?

163

The list of patients waiting for a liver transplant. What a reorganization of a worldview! She/we waited and prayed for a month.

At this point, our family had no grandfathers and two grandmothers. Her mom came at 9:00 A.M. (My day at the office had previously begun at 7:30 A.M.) Our older son got on the bus at 8:30 A.M., and our younger son got the kindergarten bus at 12:30 P.M. After four beds were made, kitchen floor swept, cat boxes cleaned, and her mom had arrived, I could leave for work. At around 12:45 P.M., my mom would arrive and take over the watch of our then 2-year-old daughter. She stayed until I got home, after visiting my wife, which was often not until between 6:30 and 7:30 P.M.

A month of this routine had passed when I received a call at 2:30 A.M. telling me a liver was available. After 19 hours in surgery, I got to see her in the surgical ICU. As I waited during those first hours of recovery to see my wife, I didn't know that this is where we would spend the next 6 months.

When school finally let out in June, I promptly took over the running of my house once again. By then my wife was finally doing so well that the surgeon was hopeful that she could be home for Father's Day. Unfortunately, a bile duct became necrotic and once again she had to be listed. We got lucky. Six days later we had another liver.

This time things went the way they were supposed to. She was able to come home at the beginning of September. Neighbors hung welcoming banners on mailboxes and front doors. The shared feeling of success/relief/gratitude was heartwarming. Although we had searched for a home with a fireplace, we hadn't been able to have more than two or three fires during the brief cold weather time she had been able to spend there. So, in an air-conditioned house with the outside temperature in the mid-90s, we had a roaring fire with her ensconced on the family room couch!

My wife had not been vertical since the preceding January. We had an occupational therapist visit twice a week to help her learn to walk again. I had converted our dining room into a bedroom for her. We also had nurses come every other day to check on her incision and my skill level at wet dressing the wound.

Within the limits of her strength and endurance, we began to live a very homey, family-oriented lifestyle. During the 4 fairly healthy years of the 5 that were granted us following the second transplant, my only outside focus was my job. While other activities were still important to us, they were just not nearly as meaningful as spending time alone or being a family together. This despite the fact that as a result of some interesting HMO exclusions, at one point we were in more than a million and a quarter dollars in debt! However, our attitude was: it's only money. You can always get more money. Just a matter of another part-time job. Where does one get another life? Another wife? Another best two-thirds of one's soul? So, we tried to reestablish what had been a fairly "traditional" home in probably what was the '60s (if not the '50s) sense of the phrase.

Without having explicitly discussed the situation very much, we decided that our kids needed as "normal" a home as was possible. We normalized. We did what we had to do without any big deal or fuss. The pervasive attitude was, "We just do what needs to be done." We didn't solicit any input regarding this. When other family members seemed to catastrophize or exaggerate, we would purposely underplay and correct later. Most people were respectful of our wishes. We never stopped living as though there would be a next year or next time. Simultaneously, she and I made a very healthy decision to stop anticipating "what will be."

From the time she had been able to come home, weekly blood tests were accepted as a matter of course. Every Monday she visited the outpatient lab at the hospital to have the level of the antirejection medication and liver enzymes checked. We'd then wait until that evening to exhale. If the enzyme levels weren't within limits, we had to be at the hospital at 7 the next morning for a liver biopsy to see what was happening. If things then went well we got to bring her home Wednesday afternoon or evening.

The first posttransplant year she spent about 50% of the time back at the hospital. Balancing the antirejection medication levels seemed tougher than it should have been. We also needed to adapt to what might be considered "corollary damage." During the 4–7 weeks following the first transplant, virtually everything that could go wrong medically did. Among other things, my wife contracted a particularly virulent strain of influenza. It did severe damage to her lungs in the context of a suppressed immune system. Several experimental medications were employed. Also necessary were a variety of antibiotics, a side effect of which was damage to the inner ear. Within a month of her homecoming, she was no longer able to use our telephone due to her hearing loss. As a result of the inner ear damage, her balance was also somewhat compromised. This, coupled with some enduring muscle difficulty finally resulted in our looking for something other than a two-story home that had all the bedrooms upstairs.

She was a coupon-clipping and garage sale-going wife who came to know very well the entire local community. She also never stopped looking for "For Sale" signs on ranch-style homes. One Sunday as I finished mowing the lawn, she returned from a search excursion and told me she had found our next house. And within hours we had bought it. Not just a house. A house close enough to ours that the kids wouldn't have to change schools. And one that included a pool.

This was October. In May we moved. It was another beginning. We felt the excitement and promise of another start, with all of the optimism, hope, and *pride this entails. We had a shared feeling that maybe we had been through the worst and a corner had been turned. We spoke of our plans for our new home and our reenergized family.*

Her Monday blood tests revealed a change in her enzyme levels. She became jaundiced. She felt ill on July 4th. Admitted to the hospital that day, she remained there for 2 weeks. Wednesday night I received a call telling me that her blood chemistry was becoming acidic and her kidneys were shutting down. She began bleeding internally. I walked with the gurney, holding her hand as she went into surgery. She never regained consciousness. When I saw her next in the ICU, her clotting factor had virtually become zero. She died Friday morning.

The next day, I went to get my kids. I asked them to join me in the backyard by the pool. The hardest thing I have ever done was to hold the three of them and tell them their mother had died.

We had planned a Florida vacation for the end of July. Determined the kids should have something besides the death of their mom to talk about when school resumed, we went. Two weeks of pure pain and loneliness.

She had been in her third new house a total of perhaps 3 weeks—not consecutively. Those plans she had time to share with me, I tried to carry out. Otherwise, I either ignored things or did what I thought she would have told me to do.

She was my wife. She managed our home, mothered our children (and me, of course), and wasn't allowed to mow the lawn or shovel the walk. I opened her car doors, pulled out her chair, investigated "noises in the dark." It's my job, it's what I do. The helplessness and frustration I felt was nothing to the overwhelming feeling of having failed in my most important role.

I was numb. I cried at least once a day for 3½ years. I also became a room mother for two of the kids, doing holiday parties and attending field trips in the best tradition of our family. I tried to retain many of the family rituals we had nourished earlier. Too soon to be comforting. I felt a little more dead every time.

Today, more than 6 years later, I have been married for nearly a year to a wonderful woman with whom I am madly in love. I am looking forward to the rest of my life with her. I am also stopped in my tracks at the most inexplicable moments by some seemingly random thought that jerks me back to a previous life. I am learning to shrug, shake it off, appreciate it, and live on. Closure? No. A wound may heal into a scar. Excruciating pain may become a dull ache. Knowledge may become wisdom. Memories that brought anguished tears may now bring a small smile. I don't think closure is an appropriate concept. It seems to imply an ending or finishing to a relationship. Some relationships will always endure. They may evolve into another order, but they will endure. To me, closure suggests a growing apart or away from someone or something. I am not certain that I can adequately label this, other than to describe a sense of depth of which I hadn't been previously aware. She will, in an indescribable way, always be part of me. One of the best parts.

—DOV

The statistics on marriage are grim. More than half end in divorce and for those who remarry, the odds that a second divorce will occur are even greater. Nevertheless, for the largest percentage of the population, marriage and remarriage continue to be the options of choice. And when couples marry they generally do so with high hopes and great expectations. Although there may be much dispute about the nature of love and whether or not couples remain together over the long term for more pragmatic and utilitarian reasons (Gottman, 1994; Lederer & Jackson, 1968), the following traditional Apache wedding blessing captures the essence both of what marriage is assumed to mean and the ideal couples seek to attain as they pledge a lifelong commitment to one another:

> Now you will feel no rain,
> for each of you will be shelter to the other.
> Now you will feel no cold,
> for each of you will be warmth to the other.
> Now there is no loneliness for you,
> for each of you will be companion to the other.
> Now you are two persons,
> but there is one life before you.
> Go now to your dwelling place,
> to enter into the days of your togetherness.
> And may your days be good and long upon this earth.

Certainly there are many marriages that endure for a lifetime that fall far short of this or any other ideal. Nevertheless, even in the midst of conflict companionship still remains. And for those whose relationships are a source of mutual satisfaction and contentment most of the time, the presence of a spouse generally means so much more. Thus, to greater or lesser degrees, a marital partner is a confidante, a person with whom one can share opinions, gossip, secrets. This is the person with whom we may feel safe enough to reveal our innermost thoughts, feelings, and fears. A spouse also may be a devil's advocate, the person who will challenge us, disagree with us, fight with us, in the security that such disagreements do not seriously threaten the relationship.

In addition, a spouse is a lover, a sexual partner, the one with whom we may share the experience of intimacy in all its dimensions. For couples with children, she or he also is the mother or father of their offspring, one's co-parent, someone with whom to share the joys as well as the trials and tribulations of childrearing. Practically, a spouse is someone who is available do to some of the driving, some of the disciplining, and some of the baby-sitting, along with a share of all of the other normal household chores.

Spouses may be advisers to one another in the areas of finances, relationships, careers, and extended family. Skilled in different areas, spouses also may be the resident painters, wallpaper hangers, repair persons, furniture refinishers, chefs, automotive experts, and gardeners. What is more, they serve as each other's "date" or escort, someone with whom to attend social gatherings, perhaps be one's bridge or bowling partner. And together spouses may enjoy a great sense of camaraderie as they share jokes, speak a private language, and understand similarly the most subtle nuances of behavior.

Also significant is the fact that a spouse often represents one's primary source of identity. Personally, she or he is the proverbial other half or best half. Often one spouse is known primarily as the husband or wife of the other. And, as a couple, spouses provide entry into a social world that many times is not open to singles. What is more, spouses are the link to each other's extended family, to grandparents, aunts, uncles and cousins, to a shared network of friendship and support.

Above all, the presence of a spouse allows for the possibility of teamwork, for a lifetime partnership. A spouse is someone with whom to grow old, someone whose very presence creates a sense of security and with whom one may share an enduring emotional bond. And when a spouse dies, it is this sense of security, which includes all the other dimensions just named, that is shattered.

However, similar to most other types of death, the actual experience of losing a spouse tends to vary considerably as a function of such circumstances as the suddenness of the dying, the gender and age of those involved, and the point in the family life-cycle stage at which the loss occurs. For example, for both widows and widowers, the most severe reactions to the death of a spouse are likely to be manifested by those who have had little or no warning. As is the case anytime death comes unannounced, the degree of pain experienced is not necessarily greater than when death is anticipated. Rather, the crucial issue is the onslaught to the coping ability of the survivor, which in this instance seems to be similar for men and women.

At the same time, women who lose a husband often report that they feel abandoned, whereas husbands tend to describe a sense of dismemberment at the loss of their wives (Kastenbaum, 1986; Zonnebelt-Smeenge & De Vries, 1998). Women generally are able to cry more freely about their loss than are men, who are more likely to behave in a manner consistent with societal constraints against the expression of emotions. Both men and women may feel angry about the death of a spouse. However, women are more likely to describe a sense of injustice and men are more likely to experience guilt.

Relative to age and family life-cycle stage, both for young couples and for those in their middle years, the death of a spouse is an occurrence out of time. In addition to the pain associated with the loss, the surviving spouse suddenly may find him- or herself the single parent of school-age or teenage children. Or, perhaps, having launched children, the couple had anticipated a new sense of freedom and the opportunity to spend more time together. By contrast, the loss of a spouse late in life, though more to be expected, also means the end of a relationship of much greater length. Thus it may be painful for very different reasons. As a recently widowed woman in her early 70s remarked soon after the death of her husband of more than 35 years, "Now I have to figure out how to live without my buddy." Indeed, the challenges of loneliness and making it on one's own are very real as remarriage becomes less likely the older the surviving spouse, which is even more probable for women than for men (Moss & Moss, 1996).

Up to this point in the introduction, we have been referring to the loss of a spouse as it typically is experienced by men and women in traditional marriages. At the same time, it is important to recognize that there are many other kinds of long-term relationships in which the death of a life partner or significant other is equivalent to the loss of a spouse. In such situations, for example, in long-term cohabitation or same-sex relationships, the loss of one member of the couple is complicated by a lack of social support for the bereaved. In addition, stigma may be part of the context because of the cause of the death, as in the case of AIDS.

Whatever the circumstance, however, many bereaved persons eventually are able to move beyond the initial pain and shock and thus find themselves desiring another committed relationship. To succeed in this endeavor, they often must face and overcome guilt, or a sense of betrayal of the deceased partner. Then they must venture into the dating arena, first finding potential partners and then dealing with feelings and situations they may not have experienced since they were adolescents or young adults. Finally, should remarriage become an option, they must cope with the ghost of the person who has died. They also may have to handle the living presence of children and the reality of stepparenting issues. Indeed, although they may change, the ramifications of the death of a spouse and the process of grieving are likely to continue for the remainder of the life of the surviving partner.

Accordingly, when the couple takes seriously the words of the marriage vow, " 'til death do us part," the loss of a spouse is one of life's most predictable occurrences. Nevertheless, no matter when the death occurs or under what conditions, it is also one of life's most stressful experiences. Indeed, according to some researchers, losing a spouse requires more adjustment than does any other life event (Holmes & Rahe, 1967). It is painful, anger-provoking, and often totally confusing. One's entire identity suddenly revolves around being an "I" rather than being both a "we" and an "I," a transition so disorienting for many that recovery may be a long and traumatic process.

To understand the various factors influencing spousal bereavement, this chapter focuses first on the similarities and differences in the way widows and widowers react to the loss of a husband or wife. Next, I consider the issue of age as well as the time in the life cycle of the family that the death occurs. The third discussion revolves around the experience of the loss of a partner in committed relationships other than marriage. And in the fourth and final section, I provide an overview of some of the challenges of dating and remarriage following the death of a spouse.

WIDOWS AND WIDOWERS

Though both may lose spouses, the death of a husband for a wife tends to be a different experience than the death of a wife for a husband. Not only the differing roles typically played by women and men but also the divergent ways in which women and men are socialized, and therefore are expected to behave, in our society are crucial to understanding the unique dimensions of grief encountered by the members of each sex. Of primary importance in this regard may be the following:

The sexes have very different languages for grief. The ways they process their emotions are unique, too. Men tend to *think* their way through grief; their intellect is their guide. Women seem to *feel* their way through grief; emotion is their pilot. So often men say they have no words to grieve with, and they describe themselves as mute. It is as if men lack a universal language to convey their feelings or clothe their experiences. They feel paralyzed. Women seem unable to get beyond their feelings. Grief overshadows their life. (Levang, 1998, pp. 15–16)

Accordingly, women are more likely to express their grief through crying (Zonnebelt-Smeenge & De Vries, 1998) and sometimes even wish they could find a way to turn off their tears (Levang, 1998). However, women do have permission to cry and generally are supported by their family members and friends to express the full range of their emotions. They may be sad. They may be angry, often at God. They also may think of the loss as completely unjust, particularly as they reflect on the positive qualities of their husbands and the life they shared together. As one widow wrote in her journal several months after the death of her husband following long-term illness:

> *It's not fair to me and the kids. R. was decent, kind, outgoing, funny, giving, handsome, cheerful, caring, willing, generous with his time.*
> *I continue to be angry at God! R. was a good, kind, generous man who always put his family first. He took good care of himself. Why did God have to deal him cancer?! He was brave; he had excellent oncology and transplant care; why couldn't those regimens cure him?!*

Despite their pain and their questioning, widows seem to cope more effectively than do widowers during the immediate aftermath of the death of a spouse. However, they tend to have more physical and emotional problems 2 to 3 years after the loss and their long-term adjustment tends to be less satisfactory (Rando, 1991). Many factors enter into the creation of such a scenario for women.

First and foremost, women tend to derive more of a sense of identity from their spouses than do men. They typically also are at greater risk financially, have more problems dealing with practical issues, and thus worry more about security for themselves and their children. They also are vulnerable because of concerns about the well-being of their children should anything happen to them as the sole remaining parents. They worry about the future and what it may hold, often feeling a lack of a sense of direction. And the future looms larger for women, who have a longer life expectancy than do men.

Socially, widows also face a much greater challenge than do widowers. There are fewer eligible men to date and often fewer ways to meet them. Moreover, women often are excluded from social gatherings because they are single and/or they are perceived as a threat to married couples. They thus may feel a decrease in self-confidence as they question whether former friends liked them only as part of a couple and not as individuals. They also may feel anger and resentment at being "dropped" by their social network. At the same time, even when included and invited to be with former friends, they may feel like a fifth wheel or the "odd man out" and thus may choose to avoid couples and couple situations. They also may wish to avoid being in the presence of sexual jokes and innuendoes. And they may resent other women who make derogatory comments about their spouses when at least they still have them.

The bereavement process for men tends to be equally painful, but the specific challenges and tendencies vary considerably. For example, husbands have been reported to experience much higher levels of distress and to suffer more physical illness, psychiatric symptomatology (Shapiro, 1994), and death following the loss of a spouse (Nolen-Hoeksema & Larson, 1999). Men also are far more likely than women to resort to suicide after the death of a wife (Walsh, 1988). These statistics are particularly relevant for widowers under the age of 75 and during the period immediately following the death of a spouse (Rando, 1991).

The dilemma for men is that they often do not have as strong a network of support as do women. And even when it does exist, they are not as likely to avail themselves of this support, at least in the realm of feelings. In addition, though men may be seen as needing greater assistance in the domestic arena, they often are treated as though they have fewer emotional needs (Zonnebelt-Smeenge & De Vries, 1998). For all these reasons, widowers tend to be more isolated than widows during the immediate aftermath of the death (Nolen-Hoeksema & Larson, 1999).

Further, given lack of familiarity with the role, men often find it more difficult than do women to take care of themselves and their households (Nolen-Hoeksema & Larson, 1999). They may be at a loss when faced with the challenges of childrearing on their own. They tend to have more problems handling even the most routine everyday tasks and responsibilities. When there are no children or the children are grown and gone, they may find that being alone is intolerable (Bouvard & Gladu, 1998).

Finally, men in our society are given messages indicating that they are supposed to be able to handle even the gravest situations. In addition, they are to do so on their own. And they certainly are not supposed to cry or make any kind of emotional display:

> Cultural pressures work to make males into "true men." Boys are taught to be strong, outspoken, and intrepid individuals, proud to bear the mantle of masculinity. Fathers, mentors, and peers define and confirm the boys' masculinity and instruct them to be independent, fearless, self-assured, and powerful. At the same time, men impress upon boys that vulnerability, tenderness, and sensitivity are weaknesses for the male gender. They give boys no names for their very real and felt emotions, and no permission to express them. (Levang, 1998, p. 27)

Unfortunately, many men have taken cultural messages such as these to heart, often to their detriment. Thus, they frequently don't spend enough time acknowledging their pain, either openly to others or privately to themselves. That is, they don't allow themselves to grieve fully. What is more, given a propensity to action, they may choose to become busy, quickly returning to work. Indeed, men typically derive a strong sense of stability and identity from their careers (Zonnebelt-Smeenge & De Vries, 1998). However, to escape the empty house and all the memories it holds, men may overwork and may stay out late. They also may not eat well and/or decide to eat the majority of their meals in restaurants (Bouvard & Gladu, 1998). Some may turn to alcohol or other drugs to assuage their pain and cope with the harsh realities of life. All these factors help to explain the poorer prognosis for men in the immediate period following the death of a spouse.

However, although more vulnerable initially, once men have managed to negotiate the first few months following the loss, they often turn much more quickly than do women to the search for a new relationship. What is more, given the greater availability of single women of all ages, men are able to find new partners much more often and to do so more rapidly (Rando, 1991). It follows, therefore, that widowers also are much more likely to remarry than are widows (Moss & Moss, 1996). And having reestablished themselves as part of a couple, husbands once again tend to see their wives as their primary support person (Shapiro, 1994). Thus it is quite likely that men, more often than women, will have someone with whom to grow old, even though they also may have experienced the death of a spouse.

As we have seen, widowhood may be quite different than widower-hood. At the same time, although gender is certainly an important con-sideration, other factors also enter into the equation for bereaved hus-bands and wives. One of these concerns the ages of the couple and the family life-cycle issues that are preeminent at the time of the death of a spouse.

THE FAMILY LIFE CYCLE

As mentioned previously, as families are created and move through time, their individual members are faced with unique developmental tasks and emotional issues relevant to each stage of the family life cycle (Barnhill & Longo, 1978; Becvar & Becvar, 2000; Carter & McGoldrick, 1980; Duvall, 1962). For the newly married young couple, the primary chal-lenge involves forming a marital system that is separate from and yet con-nected to the families of origin of the two partners. At this point in their lives, the couple also may be invested in establishing careers and creating peer relationships. Their primary focus, however, generally is on the com-mitment they have made to each other as well as the hopes and dreams they share for the future. It is a time of romance, excitement, and poten-tial.

Although it is unlikely that a spouse will die during this early period in the marital relationship, it does happen. And when it does, it may be so utterly shocking that the bereavement process is particularly traumatic for the surviving husband or wife (Parkes & Weiss, 1983). Indeed, younger spouses may be even more bereaved than older spouses (Nolen-Hoeksema & Larson, 1999). What is more, there may be little support forthcoming from peers or siblings, who often are frightened by the death or simply do not know how to respond (McGoldrick & Walsh, 1991). New in-laws also may be confused about their role or resentful when the wife or hus-band of their deceased son or daughter decides to enter into another rela-tionship. Thus, the loss of a spouse early in the marriage may be both an extremely painful and a very isolating experience.

Couples that decide to take on the responsibilities of childbearing and childrearing find themselves facing the challenges of making room in their lives both for their offspring and for the presence of grandparents.

Becoming parents also means that they have to accommodate the unique personalities of each of their children, attend to their educational and recreational needs, and deal with the increasing demands and drains on their time and energy. At the same time, they also must find ways to nurture their relationship as a couple. It is a foundational period in the life of the family.

Given the primacy of caretaking and financial obligations for families with young children, the ability of a wife or husband to mourn appropriately the death of her or his spouse may be compromised in many ways (McGoldrick & Walsh, 1991). The requirements of home, family, and work simply may not allow time for grieving. What is more, though fathers may have offers of assistance from friends and families for the handling of domestic duties, women may be perceived as not needing the same kind of help. However, being a single parent is challenging even under the best of circumstances, and despite the emotional support women otherwise may receive. The death of a spouse during the period when the children are young therefore may signal the need for various kinds of aid both to allow for grieving and to alleviate some of the family burdens.

The parents of teenagers are faced with all the challenges preparatory to launching children into the worlds of college, work, and relationships. At the same time, the members of the couple are likely to be dealing with their own midlife career and family issues, including the aging of their parents. And as they move toward the stage of the empty nest, they may have a renewed interest in and focus on their marital relationship. Described in the previous chapter as a period of turbulence and transition, it also holds promise as a time of rediscovery and recommitment for couples.

When a spouse dies at this point in time, the surviving husband or wife is left to handle on his or her own one of the most overwhelming periods in the life of any family. Further, when widowhood occurs during the middle years, it often coincides with the period during which greater freedom and financial ability might have enabled the couple to anticipate spending more time together, perhaps fulfilling dreams that previously were postponed in favor of responsibilities associated with childrearing and career considerations. Indeed, once the children leave home, the marriage often becomes the primary focus (McCullough & Rutenberg, 1988). It is thus likely that when a spouse dies in midlife, along with all the other pain and loss, spouses also will feel cheated of the time they had planned to spend together in the future (Nolen-Hoeksema & Larson, 1999).

When couples reach later life they find themselves dealing with issues associated with retirement, personal health, the support of younger generations, and the deaths of members of the older generation. Given increased life expectancy, many husbands and wives are able to enjoy a long period following retirement during which they may travel, close their family home, and move to warmer climates, often far from other family members. For many it is a period of both great satisfaction and much loss.

The death of a husband or wife is more to be expected at this point in the family life cycle, but it may mean the end of one's longest relationship, one which "involve[s] strong primary attachments that serve as a base for mutual security and protectiveness" (Moss & Moss, 1996, p. 163). Moreover, the loss may raise serious concerns not only for the bereaved person but also for other family members regarding the ability of the surviving spouse to care for him- or herself (Brown, 1988). This issue is particularly relevant for women, who are more likely than men to spend their remaining days alone. Indeed, although more predictable, the death of a spouse later in life may present issues and dilemmas that are just as significant as when the loss occurs earlier in life.

Thus, no matter what the age or stage in the family life cycle, the death of a spouse has significant ramifications far beyond the most obvious fact that a loved one has died. However, in all the situations just described, those in which the person who died was one member of a legally sanctioned marital relationship, survivors may expect and receive validation for their grief and support for their needs from the world around them. By contrast, couples in cohabitating, same-sex, or other kinds of committed relationships are much more likely to find that this is not the case.

COMMITTED RELATIONSHIPS

The choice of men and women to live together, either before or as an alternative to getting married, has become increasingly more popular over the years. The number of households with unmarried couples has grown from 439,000 in 1960 to 4.1 million in 1997 ("Singlehood & Cohabitation," 2000). Of the persons of the opposite sex who share living quarters, 58% are between the ages of 25 and 44; 21% are 45 or older; and 25% are under 25. In the 1960s, 25% of couples chose to live together before marrying. By the 1980s, this figure had risen to 70%. Therefore, it is important to recognize the prevalence of the phenomenon of cohabitation as well as the context of this particular lifestyle. That is, although the majority of heterosexual couples who live together are childless, many also bear and rear children. Indeed, cohabitation shares many similarities with marriage, including the creation of enduring emotional and physical relationships between partners of the opposite sex. What distinguishes them is the absence of the legal, religious, societal, and cultural supports afforded couples who are married.

However, cohabitation is a choice for heterosexual couples, one that may be made for a variety of reasons. By contrast, homosexual couples do not have the right to a legal marriage in the United States and thus cohabitation is their only option should they choose to live together. According to domestic partnership laws, which have been adopted only in very few areas, "same-sex partners are allowed public and legal recognition of unions which meet specified criteria, and are granted specific rights and benefits" (Rahimi, 1999, p. 2). By virtue of such laws, sick leave, hospital visitation rights, bereavement leave, and health benefits for partners, as well as financial benefits during and at the end of the relationship, are available. However, civil marriage also allows several additional benefits not available to same-sex partners even under domestic partnership rights.

Accordingly, one partner may not inherit from another without a valid will, nor may couples obtain home and automobile insurance together. They may not rent jointly, apply for immigration and residency permits for partners from other countries, or share joint custody of or have visitation rights with children, and they may not file joint tax returns, receive wrongful death benefits, have a partner covered under social security or Medicare, make medical decisions, or choose a final resting place for one another in the case of illness and/or death. Thus, like heterosexual couples who live together, few legal and societal supports exist. But for same-sex couples, these same supports are not available even if that is what they would prefer.

Other kinds of committed relationships which are not recognized, either formally or informally, are those that are secret, as with partners in extramarital affairs or in situations in which one or both members find themselves unwilling or unable to acknowledge publicly that the liaison exists. Also generally unacknowledged is the relationship between ex-spouses, which still may be intense for at least one if not both members of the couple. When the death of a partner occurs for a person in any one of a variety of committed relationships that are not socially sanctioned, the loss may be felt just as deeply as if the partners were married. However, in addition to the grief experienced, several other issues also must be kept in mind.

For example, when a relationship is not recognized, there is likely to be an absence of permission for the bereaved person to express his or her grief appropriately, perhaps even to participate in funeral and burial arrangements and ceremonies (Rando, 1991). Also, the surviving partner may lose access to the extended family of the person who has died and may be fearful of seeking help from others (Bouvard & Gladu, 1998). Compounding these factors may be guilt and/or ambivalence about the relationship as well as secrecy. In the latter case, family and friends may not even know either that the relationship existed or that the surviving partner has lost a loved one.

Further, even though public, when the relationship is between same-sex partners, the bereaved person is likely to receive little formal support, for example, to take time off from work or to inherit in a manner consistent with the wishes of the deceased. This may particularly be the case if the relationship was not approved of by extended family members on either or both sides. Indeed, "societal attitudes toward homosexuality complicate all losses in gay and lesbian relationships" (Walsh & McGoldrick, 1991, p. 23).

When the death is due to AIDS-related problems, stigma and confusion generally are added to grief: "Suicide survivors and, more recently, families with a member dying of AIDS are those whose bereavement experiences are regarded negatively, because of the assumption that the deaths were caused by the individual's disturbed or immoral behavior" (Shapiro, 1994, p. 259). It is not surprising, therefore, that gay men whose partners die of AIDS evidence high levels of depression and tend to suffer more social isolation than either the family members of their partners or the family members of people who have died from other causes (Nolen-Hoeksema & Larson, 1999).

Additional complicating factors in the case of AIDS-related deaths include the fact that those dying generally are young, their dying tends to be long and painful, and the highest percentage of such deaths occur among homosexuals, who already may feel socially isolated (Nolen-Hoeksema & Larson, 1999). What is more, within the gay community, the context of the death of a partner has been described as one of constant mourning (Shernoff, 1997), a chronic state that is complicated by, "post-traumatic stress, loss saturation, unresolved grief, survivor guilt, and fear of infection with HIV" (Dworkin & Kaufer, 1995, p. 42).

As is certainly apparent at this point, members of committed relationships whose partners die need understanding as well as support, both for the sadness experienced and for the issues that are likely to complicate the grief process. Anyone whose loved one dies feels all the pain and sadness that such a loss entails. Whether socially recognized or not, the partnerships created in committed relationships often are comparable to marriages in terms of the depth of emotion and shared hopes, expectations, and dreams. Thus, the return to normal functioning following the death of a partner may require the same time and attention as that available to widows and widowers. And, ultimately, like those whose spouse has died, the surviving partners also may find themselves facing the challenges of new relationships and new commitments.

DATING AND REMARRIAGE

Whereas thoughts of dating and remarriage initially are probably the furthest thing from the minds of those who have lost a spouse or partner, the time usually comes when the idea of venturing into this realm becomes worthy of consideration. However, it is a decision that generally requires much thought and sometimes great agonizing. For, despite the loneliness that is a part of being a widow or widower, guilty feelings, a sense of betrayal, or even the idea that one is being sacrilegious or adulterous often accompanies the prospect of creating a relationship with another man or woman (Rando, 1991; Zonnebelt-Smeenge & De Vries, 1998). In fact, "There is some evidence that widowed persons decide not to remarry in order to respect, to preserve, and not to betray their ties with the deceased spouses" (Moss & Moss, 1996, p. 169).

Nevertheless, many people eventually choose to date, and some of them remarry. As noted previously, men tend not to wait as long, nor do they worry as much about how such behavior will be perceived by others or have as much fear and anxiety about the establishment of a new relationship as do women (Zonnebelt-Smeenge & De Vries, 1998). By contrast, widows are more likely to allow at least a year to pass before beginning to date based both on feelings of loyalty toward their deceased spouse and a desire to operate in a socially acceptable manner (Moss & Moss, 1996).

In addition to waiting longer to begin, women are more likely than men to encounter difficulties in the search for someone to date. There are five times more women than men in the pool of widowed persons. Further, because widowers generally choose younger partners the second time around, there are even fewer widowers available as dating or marriage partners (Moss & Moss, 1996, p. 164). What is more, men may be reluctant to date widowed women because of the tendency of the latter to idealize their deceased spouse and the inability of a new partner to compete with such "perfection" (Lopata, 1996, p. 152).

Even when potential partners are available, however, those who decide to participate in the dating game may find the process exceedingly uncomfortable. From being in stable, committed relationships, widowed persons suddenly are plunged into a world of uncertainty and insecurity with a resurgence of feelings they may not have experienced since adolescence. They may feel awkward and unsure of themselves and also may have to confront the fact that the rules of dating, particularly around sexuality, have changed a great deal over the years.

Older people may take longer than those who are younger to find a suitable new mate, and many may choose options other than marriage to satisfy their needs. Indeed, "It seems that many people widowed in their seventies or later are not interested in remarriage. Persons in that age group may simply decide to enhance their life with good male and female friendships" (Zonnebelt-Smeenge & De Vries, 1998, p. 198). In part this may be a function of the fact that because women tend to outlive men, there are fewer available men the older one becomes. Another option more available for widowed persons today than in the past is cohabitation. Widowed people also seek to cohabitate more often because of problems around the loss of insurance and medical benefits when they remarry (Moss & Moss, 1996).

An important challenge associated with the decision to remarry is the need to be sure that what one is seeking is not just a cure for loneliness, a means to avoid grief or a replacement for the wife or husband who has died (Rando, 1991). Rather, the same considerations of compatibility in all areas that accompany a first marriage are crucial to the creation of a second marriage. Also crucial is awareness of the role that children of former marriages may play in the lives of remarried persons when one or both have been widowed.

Though surviving spouses eventually may accept the reality of the death of a husband or wife, they generally also maintain a connection with the deceased spouse and the life they shared together. Children not only represent this former relationship but tend to relate to the living parent as part of the team that included the deceased parent (Moss & Moss, 1996). Thus, the new spouse may feel threatened by the ongoing "presence" of the former relationship. It also may be difficult for the new

spouse to find a place in the family or to feel accepted by the children. Indeed, "Frequently there are problems with children who for personal or
economic reasons resent their surviving parent's involvement with someone else" (Rando, 1991, p. 133). And such problems may occur regardless
of the ages of the children.

Thus, as with other kinds of losses, the process of spousal bereavement continues long after a wife or husband dies. Widows and widowers—as well as their children and their new partners—live on in the presence of grief. Ideally, however, they are able to do so while they also find
ways to negotiate successfully the new world that emerges following the
death of a spouse.

THERAPEUTIC CONVERSATIONS
AND REFLECTIONS

∾

An adolescent male was referred to me because of school-related difficulties. A sophmore in high school, he had been having problems
since before the death of his mother, which had occurred 6 months
prior to our first meeting. Because his two older sisters were away at
college, I met only with the young man and his father. In addition to
the grief both were experiencing, the young man and his father were
in serious conflict.

Dad was a professional man in his mid-40s who was deeply concerned about his son. However, father and son had very different
orientations to the world and thus experienced great difficulty communicating effectively with one another. Dad was an engineer who
was extremely athletic, while the son's interests lay in the realms of
music and drama. Dad was a go-getter; son was rather "laid back."
Dad wanted son to follow in his footsteps. Son wanted to pursue his
own dreams. My story was that it would be important for each to
learn to respect the other and to find ways to speak in such a manner that there could be understanding between the two.

An important component of the therapy was an exploration of
the ways that each was dealing with his grief. The mother/wife had
been the cornerstone of the family as well as the peacemaker and
the buffer between the children and their father. However, though

(cont.)

she was loved by all and clearly missed, there was a strong network of support from family and friends and both son and father seemed to be managing fairly well. Indeed, what they seemed to need most was help in establishing a meaningful relationship with each other.

Also significant was the learning of more effective communication skills as well as encouragement to spend meaningful time together. Son began to share more about his feelings. As his Dad showed sincere interest, he also was able to speak more freely about his musical and theatrical interests. Dad became more willing to talk about his fears and worries, including a sense of guilt as he became involved with another woman. He also kept his son informed and included him in important decisions about his future.

Over time, the young man became more successful in school. His behavioral problems diminished and the relationship between him and his father improved dramatically. Dad was able to find ways both to express his concerns without alienating his son and to let his son know that he loved him and was proud of his accomplishments. Son was supportive of the new life his father was creating and found that the woman who had become his stepmother was a welcome source of support.

During the course of our work together, the 1-year anniversary of the death occurred. As it approached, I asked both clients how they were doing relative to any grief they might be experiencing. In the conversation that ensued, I mentioned that despite the fact that things were going well, it would not be unusual for son and father to have some more intense feelings of sadness as the date approached. I wanted them to be prepared should this happen and have found that discussing the possibility has been helpful when working with other bereaved clients. I also hoped that by anticipating this rather typical reaction, its impact might be somewhat reduced.

At the following session, I was truly taken aback when the father reported that he had been extremely angry at me for what I had said about feeling bad during our last meeting. I asked him to tell me what I had said that had angered him and he explained that he thought I had told him he *should* feel upset. At this point, the son jumped in and described his perception that what I had said was that they *might* feel upset, and that, in fact, he had experienced exactly what I had predicted. I apologized profusely for not having been clearer and assured Dad that I certainly would never attempt to give him or anyone else a problem. I explained the basis for my prediction and, fortunately, we were quickly were able to clear up the misunderstanding.

As I reflected on this experience, I was reminded, first of all, of the fact that the message sent is not necessarily the same as the message received. It is therefore always important to check out understandings and perhaps prevent possible misunderstandings. Second, it has affirmed my belief that every event is a therapeutic opportunity. As it turned out, I believe that the father and I were able to do a better job of hearing and speaking with each other after this conversation. At the same time, I also recognized that I had participated in exactly the kind of miscommunication which had been part of the presenting problem. This enabled me to be more empathic about and sensitive to the dilemma between father and son which had brought them into therapy. Finally, and perhaps most important, I understood that given the sensitivity of the issues around grief and guilt, and particularly the father's concerns about having established a new relationship so soon after his wife's death, it was doubly important for me both to be very clear about my intentions and to continue to offer affirmations about the way things were going. It also reminded me, once again, of the fact that each person's grief experience certainly is unique to that person.

CHAPTER 10

When an Extended Family Member or Friend Dies

‿

Several strong feelings were evident to me when my youngest brother's oldest child, who was just 3 years old, was diagnosed with stage 4 neuroblastoma cancer. These feelings were consistently present throughout his nearly 2½-year treatment phase, his 3½-month dying phase, and certainly after his heart-wrenching death. First, I felt guilty that cancer had struck one of my brother's children and not one of mine. My family and I, although affected deeply by this experience, were able to continue on with our lives on a daily basis. We maintained our regular work, school, and home schedules. At one level, it felt as though the cancer had not touched us and I was both grateful for that and felt guilty at the same time.

Another equally strong, and very tangible, feeling I had was helplessness. I have always, since I was very little, been a person who gained comfort, purpose, and value through being able to help others or to contribute something of value. I am my brother's oldest sister. I had diapered and fed him as a baby and here I was in a situation where he and his family were in a tremendously painful and vulnerable place and I didn't have the slightest idea what they needed or how I could be of help to them.

What both complicated and helped the situation was that my brother and his wife and family had an incredible support system. They were inundated with their friends and his wife's family members. All were quickly filling in all the spaces and positions of obvious need. All meals were prepared and delivered, round-the-clock child care was offered for their other children, and plans were always in process to entertain and distract my nephew from his painful and ever-present cancer.

As much as I was his sister and was closely connected to my brother and his family, I still wasn't as close, on a daily and practical level, as his friends, my parents, and his wife's family. I felt I was more of an outsider from that perspective. I didn't want to compete with all the efforts being offered to them, and yet, I couldn't imagine being his sister, and living so close to them, without doing something to show my love and support. The question was, what?

During the earlier stages of this experience, I happened to meet and talk with a friend I hadn't seen in years. This friend had lost his youngest child about a year before. I felt so fortunate to be able to chat with him openly and honestly about my brother's son and about my own struggle with how to help the family. I asked him what had been especially helpful, and even unhelpful, during the death and dying of his daughter. He reconfirmed that when he had been asked by friends and family about what they could do to help, he simply hadn't been able to say at the time. Because he was so absorbed in his role as a primary caregiver to his dying daughter, he couldn't get enough of a perspective to be able to tell others how they could be of assistance.

What he ultimately found to be helpful was when others would see a need and take care of it, respectfully, but simply through action. He recounted how someone had made a point of gathering all their dirty laundry and returning it, washed and folded. Another person even came to their home and went around polishing all their shoes. Still another person made sure they were stocked with the basic grocery essentials.

This was the bit of information I needed and it helped me to sift through what I enjoy doing the most and would feel most authentic in offering to my brother and his family. I say "authentic" because I wanted whatever I did to come from who I am and what I believe. So after thinking, and even praying about it, I decided to do a few specific, rather simple things that I think offered some comfort and let them know that I was there, loving and supporting them. Because I am a strong believer in a regular, healthy diet, especially when someone is feeling stressed and drained, I occasionally brought a bag of groceries. My ordinary offerings filled in around the many spectacular dinners and breakfast treats that were a constant flow into their home. I provided fresh fruits and vegetables, milk, bread, cereal, and the like. It was a relief to have found something I could do, a place where I could fit.

Another thing I did was become the "story lady." On occasions when we were to be together as a large family, I selected several books from a wonderful children's collection I had been building over the years. I would gather any interested children in our extended family (our children and all of my brother's children, including my nephew when he felt up to it) and let them pick from the colorful pile of young children's books. As long as even one child wanted to listen, I would read. I will always treasure those moments because they were so soothing and peaceful. The storybooks allowed us, if only briefly, to forget the tragedy we were living.

All the things we did for my brother's family during this long painful journey were simple, very practical, and always nurturing. I was grateful to have figured out how to do something, no matter how small or infrequent, that fit somewhere in the larger picture of loving and supporting. This helped to relieve my feelings of guilt and helplessness.

My nephew's death has had a profound effect on me and my family. He was a small child of just barely 6 at the time he died and had been living and struggling with the cancer for nearly 3 years. The death of a relative is difficult, but the loss of a young child to such a painful disease is almost unbearable. This experience was further confounded by the fact that this was the child of my youngest sibling—the "baby" of our family. In addition, my nephew was named after my brother, who was named after my father. So, with his death, the patriarchal name also died. All these factors contributed to the feeling that life had gone terribly awry.

During the process of hoping, praying for healing, and finally accepting the reality that my nephew would not survive this cancer, we came to some helpful realizations. The obvious recurring questions that kept nagging at us were, "Why a child?" and "Why one with so much promise and possibility for the future?" It didn't seem to make any sense and, of course, it didn't make sense as long as we continued to believe that my nephew was robbed of his chance to live a full life.

I finally found peace in a simple but profound personal revelation. That is, life in its fullness comes in many different lengths. It is we who have decided that we all must live to a ripe old age, where we will see our children's children. I have now come to believe that it is possible to live a complete and full life in what feels to us an unjustly small amount of time. Some people are blessed with the ability to offer so much in a relatively brief time span.

Of course, not everyone in our extended family, especially my nephew's mother and father, would easily attach to this idea and I'm not sure I would have been able to embrace this mental and emotional shift if a child of mine had died. Nonetheless, I feel fortunate to have had enough distance from this tragedy to have gained this new perspective.

I did not share this revelation with my brother and his wife. I did share it, however, with friends, my parents, my husband, and my own children, who were 9, 7, and 4½ at the time of my nephew's death. I also felt it was important to use the moment as an opportunity to teach our children about death as a part of life. I wanted to help them see the end of our physical life as something that has purpose and meaning, even though it breaks our hearts. Still, it was difficult to know at the time what our children's experience of all this was.

Throughout all of my nephew's sickness, dying, and death, my husband and I made a point of answering any of our children's questions openly and honestly. Two years later we had an opportunity to get a glimpse of how this experience had touched one of our children. Our oldest child, who was in the fifth grade then, was given an assignment to write a "chapter book." She decided to write her book about her cousin and his death. At this point, she was 11 and was able to look back at her experience with more reflection and understanding. In her story she recounted what she had felt as a child, and as a cousin, watching another child struggle with sickness and finally die. Her simple, honest words were striking and profound. She wrote a conclusion in her final chapter that summed up what she had learned from this experience. She said: "It seems that my cousin knew how to take life one day at a time. Maybe that's what I've learned from him, that his life was going so slowly that he got more out of life in six years than most of us would ever have gotten in a normal lifetime. . . . I'd like to encourage people to try to think about life, one day at a time."

I think, for all of us, we have learned that life is not guaranteed. It is a gift, every single day. We treasure family moments in a special way now. We always say prayers to my nephew, light candles on holidays, and anniversaries and mention his name openly and frequently at family gatherings. He has become our personal family patron saint on whom we rely to help us find lost items, endure scary moments, and manage difficult situations. We feel privileged to have our own little angel watching over us and we celebrate his "angel birthdays" on the anniversary of his death.

Guided and taught by my brother and his wife, we have all come to appreciate my nephew's brief but profound life and marvel at the unending ramifications that his life and death had, and still have, on us all. We do not take things for granted now but often make a point of expressing our gratitude for things, both marvelous and simple.

Of course, this is not the complete story, but it is a good beginning of the story of how the experience of the death of my nephew has touched and influenced my life and that of my family.

—BMM

Despite the emphasis within our culture on individualism and autonomy, all our lives are lived in the context of relationships. We are born into and grow up in families of one kind or another. In addition to parents and siblings, we also may be fortunate enough to have an assortment of grandparents, aunts, uncles, and cousins—some related by blood, others not. When we enter school, we are surrounded by classmates and teachers and thus we enter the realm of friendships. We participate in sports, musical ensembles, and various other activities with teammates and friends who share our interests. We graduate from high school and college in cohorts and celebrate each other and our achievements at class reunions. A maid or matron of honor as well as a best man serve as witnesses at our marriages and the attendants who comprise our wedding parties generally also include friends and relatives of both bride and groom.

What is more, as children, even when we have been blessed with close-knit families and meaningful and supportive connections with parents and siblings, we may form special relationships with an extended family member or friend. And in instances in which parents and/or siblings may not have met our needs, an aunt or uncle, a grandparent, perhaps a teacher, may play a vital role in our development and our ability to succeed. In addition, as adults in a highly mobile society, one in which family members may be scattered across the country or the world, we also may find that friends have become our "chosen" families. These are the people with whom we celebrate holidays, share important occasions, and turn to for support in times of need. Indeed, some of our most important relationships may be formed with those outside our immediate families.

Though the bonds we form with extended family members, as well as those with family members, may wax and wane in intensity over the years and friends certainly may come and go, we generally have a few special people with whom we remain close, at least in memory if not in fact. What is more, life in the work world also inevitably offers us colleagues and coworkers with whom we share large portions of our daily lives if not our deepest emotional attachments. Together we create routines and establish identities by means of which we come to know ourselves and each other.

Another type of relationship that may be extremely important is the one formed with pets. For many people, a dog, a cat, a rabbit, or any one of a variety of animals become companions that share a connection characterized by unconditional love. For those who have experienced such a relationship, pets may be as much, or more, a part of the family than are human members. Pets often have shared a long history with their owners, they have provided comfort for one another and the love and affection experienced between them may go as deep as that between humans. In such instances, pets truly have fulfilled the position of best friend.

Considering for a moment only human loss, despite the roles that various people may play in our lives and the places they may hold in our hearts, when a person dies the significance of the event in the eyes of others generally is based on the degree of the kin relationship. For example, absence from work to attend a funeral generally is granted when a child dies or in the cases of parental and sibling loss. Rarely is the same consideration given to the death of an extended family member such as an aunt, uncle, or cousin, and almost never is the loss of a friend so recognized (Rando, 1991). Indeed, similar to situations described in the previous chapter, we once again may be confronted with a lack of recognition of or social validation for the grief experience when an extended family member or friend dies.

That is, close family members of the deceased may not acknowledge or even be aware of the depth of grief being experienced by those outside their immediate circle (Smith, 1996). At the same time, extended family members and friends who are grieving deeply internally may refrain from external expressions for fear of intruding on the immediate family. Coworkers who lose a colleague may be totally confused about how to behave with one another. They may be unable to attend the funeral or other rituals. They also may be wary of speaking about the person who has died and may find little support for their grief. And the parents of a child who has experienced the death of a classmate may not understand the impact of such a loss or take appropriate steps to deal with its ramifications.

Returning now to the possibility that the best friend who died was an animal, we find perhaps an even greater lack of understanding. Many simply do not comprehend what it means to be connected to a pet and others who have a pet may not be as deeply attached. Thus, if one admits to unbearable grief over the death of an animal, the response of others may be disbelief at best and laughter or ridicule at worst.

Indeed, we may do a grave disservice, however inadvertent, when we fail to consider the nature of the relationship between people or between a person and an animal in addition to the degree of biological connection between the deceased and others in her or his world. That is, the impact of the death of an extended family member or friend—whether soul mate, coworker, classmate, or pet—is likely to vary as a function of the level of closeness experienced by the survivor with the one who has died. In the case of a human death, relevant factors include the role played by the deceased person and his or her perceived importance, as well as whether or not there was emotional dependence between them (Brown, 1988). Other considerations of significance include the ages of those involved as well as the implicit messages sent and received by the timing of the death. Unresolved issues and ambiguity in the relationship with the person who has died also may influence the grief process. In the case of an animal death, factors of importance include the length and depth of the relation-

ship, the presence or absence of other sources of support in the life of the
pet owner, and sensitivity to the way in which the death occurred.

To understand more fully how a death may reverberate far more
broadly than often is acknowledged, the major topics of consideration
in this chapter include, first, the varieties of bereavement that may be
experienced by those who have lost an extended family member. This
topic is followed by an examination of what it means to have a close
friend die and how this event may differ in significance at various times
in our lives. This chapter then turns to the impact on colleagues of the
death of a coworker, with a particular focus on ways that the system as a
whole may be affected. Next, I consider the death of a classmate both
for young children and for adolescents. Finally, I explore the relationship that may exist between a human being and an animal and the grief
that may follow the death of a pet. In each case, as always, the goal is
to increase our ability to provide meaningful support in the presence of
grief. However, in this instance the need above all is for increased sensitivity and awareness when the one who has died is an extended family
member or friend.

DEATH OF AN EXTENDED FAMILY MEMBER

We tend to think of the large extended family with several generations either living together under one roof or in close proximity to one another as
a phenomenon of the past. Certainly relative to the frequency of such arrangements in earlier eras there is much truth in this perception and certainly it does indeed apply to many families today. But despite the overall
change in demographics over time relative to this dimension, many tight-
knit family groups still continue the pattern of remaining close to home
and comprise the basic source of support for one another. And even when
adult children move away from the family home and perhaps are scattered
in various locations, a relative such as an uncle or a grandparent may become a permanent resident or a regular visitor in one or more of these
households. Thus, although the form may vary, the extended family is often very much alive and well and relationships within it may be extremely
important.

In addition, although the traditional extended family may no longer
be the norm, family configurations are likely to be significantly influenced
as a function of ethnicity. For example, much research has enabled us to
understand the black family as a cultural variant (Allen, 1978) with a dis-

tinctive African heritage (Ladner, 1973; D. K. Lewis, 1975; Mathis, 1978; Nobles, 1978). Typically it is characterized by an extensive kin network which provides both economic and emotional support to its members (Billingsley, 1968; Gutman, 1976; Hill, 1971; Martin & Martin, 1978; McAdoo, 1980). Given the importance of the black extended family, which includes both kin and "fictive" kin relationships and often reaches across great geographical distances, the death of one of its members may have a tremendous impact, one that cannot be measured solely by blood-lines. Thus we are reminded of the following:

> There are several . . . issues to keep in mind when working with African-American families around issues of death and mourning. One cannot make assumptions about the meaning of a death simply on the basis of immediacy of the relationship; a relationship with a member of the extended family may hold as great or greater significance for an individual than a relationship with a member of the nuclear family. (McGoldrick et al., 1991, p. 191)

Of major importance, of course, is the reminder to avoid making an assumption about the grief that anyone may be experiencing. Each person is unique and we can never know, unless we are willing to probe more deeply, how important the relationship may have been. Similarly, an assessment of the broader context often is required to fully understand the ramifications of the death of an extended family member.

To illustrate, I am reminded of woman in her early 30s who came to therapy because of a variety of physical symptoms as well as an inability to form a lasting, committed relationship. As part of my initial effort to gather information I learned that she was the oldest of seven children, that her parents had remained married despite ongoing hostilities that began far back in her childhood, and that she had had a particularly conflicted relationship with her mother. Her refuge had always been an older second cousin, with whom she had remained close over the years and who recently had died after a brief illness.

The death of my client's cousin, by itself, was an extremely painful loss. To make matters worse, however, her mother and her cousin had never gotten along and her mother had always resented the bond between her daughter and the other woman. My client's siblings also were jealous of the close relationship between their older sister and their cousin. Following the cousin's death, the mother continued to make derogatory comments about her, even blaming her for her death because she had not taken appropriate care of herself. And very little sympathy for the loss was forthcoming from either my client's father or her brothers and sisters, nor did they share similar feelings of deep affection for the woman who died.

My client had thus lost the person whom she thought of as her real mother. She was bereft and felt a great void in her life. What is more, few of her friends had any idea about the extent of the loss when she reported that her sadness was due to the fact that her cousin had died. And in addition to a general lack of validation for what she was experiencing, the people to whom she might most logically think of turning—her family of origin—not only were unable to provide support but, in fact, behaved in a manner that exacerbated her grief.

Clearly, step one in the process of healing involved allowing my client to tell her story and listening to it in such a manner that she felt truly understood and that her responses were deemed appropriate. Step two included finding ways in which she could express her grief appropriately and take time to allow herself to mourn. Step three focused on learning how to let her friends know both what was really going on and what they could do to help her. Step four aimed at ways both to have realistic expectations about the kind of support her family members could provide and to establish boundaries that would enable her to feel safe when she was in their presence. As each of these steps was accomplished, the physical symptoms began to diminish and ultimately disappeared. What is more, by the end of therapy the promise of a lasting, committed relationship was looming large.

Grief thus can take many forms and the source of the pain may not be immediately obvious, particularly when the individual who died was not a member of the bereaved person's immediate family. For example, as others also have noticed, "In our experience, the death of a grandparent is often an underlying precipitant when parents seek treatment for their adolescent's problem behavior" (McGoldrick & Walsh, 1991, p. 42). Or, perhaps, the death was one more in a series of losses that eventually have become overwhelming. Careful and sensitive exploration of the larger context are thus always in order in the case of the death of an extended family member. And certainly this also holds true in situations in which the person who died was a close friend.

DEATH OF A CLOSE FRIEND

Just as the death of an extended family member may have a greater impact than the loss of a member of one's family of origin, so also may we grieve the death of a close friend even more deeply than we do the death of a family member to whom we are closely related by blood (Rando, 1991). Indeed, we may find many instances throughout history in which the importance of friendship and the significance of the loss of a friend is noted. For example, according to the Roman philosopher, dramatist, and statesman Seneca, "Next to the encounter of death in our own bodies, the most sensible calamity to an honest man is the death of a friend; and we are not in truth without some generous instances of those who have preferred a friend's life before their own" (in Woods, 1957, p. 227).

What is more, for a variety of reasons friendships today seem to have grown in significance. The most obvious source of change is the increased mobility in our society and the fact that family members are not as likely to live near one another. And even in situations in which distances are small and relationships are close, we may find those who are more inclined to do their deepest sharing with friends. This may be the case particularly for the growing number of young people who choose to remain single rather than marry and for whom friendships take on additional meaning (Bouvard & Gladu, 1998). And for those who lack attachment to families of origin, the friendships which evolve into deep and lasting relationships may become that much more precious. According to one observation relative to this phenomenon:

> Americans have great difficulty initiating and nurturing friendships given the "here today, gone tomorrow" mentality that is so prevalent in our mobile culture. In an epidemic of dysfunctional families, many of us are hungry, if not desperate, for meaningful friendships. Among the young and the elderly, friendship is emerging as the valued relationship in our culture. Many people are closer to friends than to family; friends become *de facto* families. (Smith, 1996, p. 14)

However, there may be a gender difference relative to the issue of friendship (Smith, 1996), although for both men and women the death of a close friend may be deeply felt. As noted in Chapter 9, men are likely to see their wife as their main source of support and to have few nonspouse friends. Perhaps because of the requirements of friendship to be vulnerable and to share deeply, perhaps because of fears based on homophobic beliefs, men differ from women, who often form many close friendships. However, the one or two close relationships with friends that men are likely to create tend to become extremely important and the loss of such a relationship leaves a great void. Women, by contrast, are at risk by virtue of the fact that they are so good at forming relationships. That is, they, "tend to create rich social networks and have better friendship skills—evident in both making and nurturing friendships. Because of this, women are far more vulnerable in relationships" (Smith, 1996, p. 15).

Regardless of their number, friends are the special people whom we have specifically chosen to be in our lives. They have stuck with us through the bad times as well as the good. We have been mentors, teachers, and sounding boards for one another. We have a history together. Although we may move apart, we remain close. When a friend dies we feel lost, confused, empty. What is more, our friends are generally of the same or similar age. Thus, the death of a friend reminds us of our own humanness as well as our frailties and vulnerabilities (Bouvard & Gladu, 1998).

For example, if we are both in early adulthood, we may find it hard to accept and understand the death of our friend. We generally have had little experience in this area. We may feel threatened. We may wonder why it is the friend who has died and whether we will be next. And we certainly don't expect a person who is as young as we are to die.

The loss of friends becomes a more common occurrence as we move into middle age. Although it is thus less shocking, it becomes a continual reminder of our own mortality. In addition, it is typical at this age to begin to think more in terms of the time until death rather than the time since birth (Eisdorfer & Lawton, 1973). Thus, each death is likely to trigger reflections about the meaning of life and the relatively short period of time we are granted in this reality.

When we lose a friend during the later years, it is likely to be part of the ongoing shrinking of our social network. At this point in life, "Losing a friend means losing yet another thread which connects us to the world. When our parents are gone, a friend may be the last person who shared our memories and histories" (Bouvard & Gladu, 1998, p. 120). At the same time, there may be a devaluing by others of the meaning of the loss because the person was old, or had lived a good life, the implication being that it was OK for that person to die.

Similar messages are likely to be received, at any age, if the friend who died carried in life a stigma of one sort or another. For example, "If your friend was mentally ill, physically disabled, HIV-positive, homeless, old, a criminal, or was an alcoholic or a substance abuser, our society can subtly imply that this individual did not count and we shouldn't grieve" (Smith, 1996, p. 16). Indeed, for the same reasons we may be reluctant to speak of our loss or share the depth of our grief when such a person dies.

Additional complicating factors when a friend dies include the fact that we may have been excluded from information regarding an impending loss, we may have refused to acknowledge the severity of the diagnosis, or we may have received news of the death after the fact. Perhaps because we lived at a great distance from one another we were not able to visit during an illness or we were denied visiting privileges because we were not part of the immediate family. Perhaps we were unable to attend the funeral because of either logistics or work constraints. Perhaps it has taken time for us to understand the depth of our feelings and the significance of the loss. For these and other reasons, the following advice is therefore offered:

> Grieve!!! Because no one encourages you, as a friend, to grieve. Because you may have been halfway across the country when your friend died, you did not get to participate in the rituals. Because your employer probably had no provisions in personnel policies allowing you to attend rituals for friends. Because no one sent you a "thinking of you" card or telephoned with a word of encouragement. Because no one recognizes your lingering, unshakable grief. Because you have grieved or are now grieving alone. (Smith, 1996, p. 9)

Such admonitions also have relevance even in instances in which the relationship with the friend who died was less intense. Thus, we now turn our attention to losses in two important subsets of friends. The first are those who, as adults, are our colleagues or coworkers. The second are those who are our classmates during the period in which we are young children or we are adolescents.

DEATH OF A COLLEAGUE OR COWORKER

For those employed outside the home, the highest percentage of their waking hours are likely to be spent at their places of business or on the job. Over time, it is not at all unusual for strong relationships to develop between colleagues and coworkers. Such relationships may encompass both business-related interactions and the sharing of personal information. Some may develop into important friendships that extend well beyond working hours. And even in cases in which the relationships are not deeply personal, a sense of stability may be created through familiarity with both predictable personalities and stable routines. It is therefore not surprising that a death in the workplace of someone known and perhaps greatly respected may have serious implications for those who must return to their jobs and face the void thus created.

It is quite predictable that deaths will occur among those who work together for any length of time. However, as with the loss of a friend who is close in age, the death of a colleague or coworker often means that someone in our peer group has succumbed. Hitting very close to home, "the death of a co-worker no matter what the cause or circumstances, is always premature; it reminds those in good health that life is not forever and that mortality is fleeting and forces them to consider the impending reality of their own deaths" (Nurmi & Williams, 1997, p. 43).

In addition, certain kinds of death may have a more traumatic effect on colleagues and coworkers than do others (Nurmi & Williams, 1997). These include instances in which the death occurred as a result of murder or suicide, was sudden and unexpected, or took place in the line of duty. Another potentially traumatizing factor may be the belief among coworkers that the death was due to employer negligence and thus could have been prevented. However, even when death followed a long illness or was the result of natural causes, a variety of normal grief reactions on the part of the individual survivors certainly is to be expected.

What is more, such a death may have a significant impact on the workplace environment as a whole. Depending on the role of the deceased in the larger organization of social relationships, his or her absence may lead to great stress and tension or, in extreme cases, to the breakdown of this network (Williams & Nurmi, 1997). And, in other cases, although the relationship with the person who died was not intense, the ramifications may be worthy of consideration. For example, the loss of a friendly greeting, perhaps a slap on the back, on a regular basis may seriously undermine a stable pattern and thus one's sense of self in that place (Smith, 1996).

At the same time, the typical and certainly understandable response generally made by employers is to emphasize the need to carry on and to complete business as usual. That is, the workplace generally cannot afford to risk a lapse in productivity. Therefore, colleagues and coworkers must continue to work despite their grief. In addition, the workload of the one who has died must be parceled out and taken over. And, in many cases, an office or other work space must be cleaned out and perhaps reassigned. All these factors may increase the distress felt by the survivors.

The aftershocks of such deaths also may reverberate throughout various other systems. For example, the ability of the bereaved to function normally, not only at work but also at home or in other settings, may be seriously challenged. However, family members and friends may not understand what is going on or know how to respond appropriately to the person who is grieving. Further, the bereaved colleague or coworker may not be able to articulate the dimensions of the loss or describe, even to him- or herself, exactly what is being experienced, especially if such feelings—which may include confusion, chaos, pain, dismay, and/or devastation—are new or come as a surprise.

To provide assistance in situations in which a death has taken place in the workplace, we can help to normalize the experience by explaining that the reactions being felt are both predictable and understandable. Family members and friends can be given information which enables them to have a more complete sense of what is happening and thus do a better job of supporting the grieving person. The grieving coworkers and colleagues can be helped to recognize how the change in context created by the death will inevitably impact everyone in that context.

In addition, employers can be encouraged to respond with sensitivity and consideration despite the need for continued productivity. Accordingly, small alterations in the arrangement of facilities may make the absence of the person who has died less obvious. Further, provision may be made for counseling or for support group meetings among the remaining employees.

Regardless of the circumstances of the death, it is important to remember the potential for healing that may be supported or undermined by the response of an organization to the death of an employee and the impact it has on colleagues and coworkers: "If a death is ignored, if a deceased employee is quickly replaced (as if forgotten), or if persons grieving a death are isolated or discounted, secondary reactions are more likely to develop. Working in a caring, people-oriented environment contributes to resistance to traumatic stress. Thus the habitual patterns of interaction of an organization may influence the healing of its employees greatly" (Williams & Nurmi, 1997, p. 195).

Indeed, as with families, the loss of one of the members in a workplace setting affects not only each individual but also the system as a whole. And, conversely, the healing of the system is facilitated to the extent to which each person is responded to with sensitivity and understanding. In a similar manner, we also may recognize the importance of creating a caring, people-oriented environment in order to help alleviate the pain that children or adolescents may experience when a classmate dies.

DEATH OF A CLASSMATE

During the course of the many years spent in school, children often are faced with the death of a classmate as the result of either illness or an accident. From time to time, natural disasters such as earthquakes and tornadoes also may create tragedies when schools or classmates become victims. Certainly these are not new phenomena and fortunately they do not occur with great regularity. However, in an era in which violence appears to be on the increase everywhere, it is important to be aware of the fact that today more and more children are being exposed to the death of schoolmates at an early age (Nader, 1997b), and often these deaths have occurred in a brutal and potentially traumatizing manner.

Indeed, several occurrences involving the murder of a number of children, often by older students attending the same school, have received national attention in the news media. In addition, all too often we may read or hear about one child being killed by another either in or out of school. Drive-by and accidental shootings also may take the lives of classmates as well as others in the world of children. For example, in a recent incident in St. Louis, a beloved fifth-grade teacher was shot to death at a shopping mall one week prior to the opening of the school year.

Also on the increase is the incidence of suicide among young people. According to one set of statistics, the rate of suicide among young men ages 15 to 24 tripled between 1955 and 1980 and more than doubled for young women in the same age group during this same period (Hendin, 1995). What is more, suicide now accounts for 8% of deaths among those ages 5 to 19 (U.S. Public Health Service, 2000), and among teenagers it is the third leading cause of death after accidents and homicide (National Center for Health Statistics, 1996). In fact, "Suicide haunts our literature and our culture. It is the taboo subtext to our successes and our happiness. . . . Yet suicide happens every day, and many people we know have had a relative or a friend who has committed suicide" (Shneidman, 1996, p. 4). And as difficult and painful as it is for adults to understand and accept, suicide may be even more puzzling and disorienting for children and adolescents.

When a classmate dies, support becomes necessary within systems such as a school the child attended or where the death occurred. Family members also must be alert to the importance of sensitivity to the potential impact of the experience and the specific needs of children or adolescents. Specialized methods of trauma treatment may be required depending on the nature of the death and the degree of involvement of the survivors:

> When there is a traumatic death, a child who is affected must contend with the symptoms of trauma, of grief, and of the interaction between the two. The response to traumatic death is further complicated by the fact that catastrophic events can effect entire communities. An entire family, classroom or group, school or agency, or community may grieve over the traumatic loss of one or more individuals. (Nader, 1997b, p. 159)

Following noncatastrophic loss, children typically experience such reactions as yearning and/or searching; reminiscing; grief dreams; grief play; somatic reactions; and distressing thoughts. When the death occurs under traumatic circumstances children are likely to be challenged as well by questions about why the event occurred; intrusive and distressing recollections; traumatic or bad dreams; traumatic play or reenactment; somatic reactions; and intense distress in response to reminders of the event (Nader, 1997a). In the case of suicide among young people, surviving classmates also may find themselves utterly confused and conflicted by what has taken place. The death is both sudden and the result of a conscious choice on the part of the one who has died. It thus was preventable. Given its deliberate nature, "this act fuels intense feelings of rejection, abandonment, and desertion in those left behind. This can contribute to a profound shattering of your self-esteem, with strong feelings of unworthiness, inadequacy, and failure" (Rando, 1991, pp. 111–112).

Although such reactions are likely to be more intense for those most closely related to the person who has committed suicide, classmates are highly vulnerable as well. What is more, if the death is one in a series of losses, grief reactions are likely to be more severe. Thus, when a classmate dies, children and adolescents require and deserve the sensitive support and knowledgeable understanding of others in their world. The same may also be said, and regardless of age, for those who have lost a pet with whom they shared a close relationship.

DEATH OF A PET

Recent encounters with two different clients have reinforced for me an awareness of the degree of grief people may feel when a pet dies. In the first instance, a middle-age man was absolutely incensed by the perceived insensitivity of his younger brother to the death of his dog. Although his other siblings and several friends had expressed their condolences either through cards or loving messages delivered in person or over the telephone, this particular brother had done nothing. My client took this lack of sensitivity as a personal affront and will be hard-pressed to forgive the oversight even if apologies are forthcoming in the future.

In the second instance a woman in her early 30s who was recently divorced was wrestling with a decision about whether to allow her seriously ailing dog to be put to sleep. In addition to all the moral and ethical questions about euthanasia, she also was plagued by several other concerns. Thus, she was struggling with the fact that she and her pet had shared much together, that the dog's death would mean the deprivation of her closest companion, that it would signify with utter finality the end of the era that included her marriage, and that it was yet one more in a series of losses.

Having had similar experiences with a much loved dog who died after 15 years of shared history, I was able to empathize with my clients. However, unless they also are animal lovers, others often are quite unsympathetic to what it may mean to lose a pet. Offhand comments about the fact that it was "just" a dog, cat, bunny, and so on, and therefore can be replaced easily, are among the most typical responses to such a death. Unfortunately, not only are comments such as these insensitive, but they also may exacerbate the grief of the person whose pet has died.

Indeed, such a loss may be overwhelming for it means the severing of what has been termed the human–companion animal bond (Rosenberg, 1986). And such bonds may go very deep:

> "As every pet owner knows—and close to 60 percent of all households in the United States include a cat or a dog—animals can be more loyal, more cuddly, and infinitely less critical than people. Our relationships with cats and dogs can also last twenty years or more—longer than many marriages— and during that time, our pet loves us unreservedly" (Lightner & Hathaway, 1990, pp. 176-177).

Nevertheless, there is a general lack of social recognition when a pet dies. Not only are there no publicly approved rituals, but when a person chooses to have a funeral or other ceremony for a pet, he or she often is faced with derision, or at least lack of understanding. But those who are mourning the death of a pet deserve to be taken seriously (O'Maley,

2000). Their grief is real and the pain they are experiencing is worthy of as much care and consideration as we would offer anyone who is hurting.

Indeed, the basic theme running throughout this chapter is the need for awareness of the emotional upheaval that may be created for others in our world by a death, especially when it may not appear on the surface to constitute a significant loss. Those who have lost an extended family or friend may be mourning the end of one of the most important relationships in their lives. As we are able to recognize the degree of grief in whose presence these others may be living, we may do them, as well as ourselves, a great favor.

THERAPEUTIC CONVERSATIONS
AND REFLECTIONS

∿

A high school counselor was alerted by concerned teachers that one of the top students in the senior class, a 17-year-old female, had suddenly begun to have trouble completing homework assignments and that her test grades had dropped significantly. As the end of the year and graduation were not far off, they at first thought that "senioritis" had set in. However, further questioning revealed that the young woman was deeply troubled and might benefit from counseling.

After a lengthy exploratory conversation with the student, the counselor spoke to the young woman's parents and requested that they seek family therapy. What the counselor had learned, and what ultimately was shared with me, was a story of loss and grief that were seriously impeding the ability of the young woman to concentrate. Although the parents were also grieving, and had knowledge of some of the extenuating circumstances, they had not been fully aware of what had been transpiring for their daughter, who was an only child.

About a year prior to our meeting, the young woman's grandmother, her father's mother, who had lived with the family since early in her parent's marriage, had died after a long and painful illness. Grandmother and granddaughter had been very close, so her

(cont.)

loss left a great empty space in the house, both physically and emotionally. What is more, she had died at home and the young woman had watched her gradual decline as well as her death. Although both the parents and their daughter were thus deeply saddened, they all seemed to have been recovering rather well. And so they were.

However, a classmate of the young woman had recently committed suicide. They were not close friends, but she and many other students were stunned by the death of one of their peers, a young woman who was popular and seemed to have a great deal going for her. For the young woman who was my client, not only was this second loss extremely upsetting but it also triggered flashbacks of the death of her grandmother. She found herself picturing again how her grandmother had suffered and was reliving repeatedly the moment of her death. Although she knew that it was important to do better in school, she had been unable to study and then had become more upset when her efforts to do so were unsuccessful. What is more, she had been reluctant to share with her parents what was going on for fear of making them sadder than they already were about the death of the grandmother.

After listening to their stories and getting a sense of what might be happening, I encouraged each of the members of this family to share and discuss with one another their ideas about what happens after death. During the course of this conversation we also talked about other losses that each person had experienced as well as the way each had chosen to deal with the grief. In addition, we explored the recovery process related specifically to the death of the grandmother and what they as a family had been doing to honor her memory.

Then, with the family's permission, I contacted and began to work with the school counselor, who agreed to inform all the young woman's teachers about what was going on. Because it was near the end of the year and the young woman was a good student, arrangements were made that allowed for the postponement or cancellation of her exams. The young woman also was given permission to leave class should she feel the need.

Indeed, I encouraged the young woman to allow herself whatever time and space she required to feel sad and to understand that mourning is not a time-limited process. I suggested that she start writing about her thoughts and feelings in a journal. I invited the family to spend time together periodically going through all their old photographs and to create a memorial album of the beloved grandmother. As they worked on the album I also invited them to share both their images and their memories of the many happy times they had spent together. And I explained my belief in the importance of being able to talk openly about dying, death, and what comes after.

I believe that the young woman whose story I have just described was extremely fortunate to have been going to a school in which the staff were able to be so alert and responsive in a positive manner to the needs of their students. She also was blessed with caring and sensitive parents who were willing and able to pursue therapy. Although the feelings of mutual love and concern added to the young woman's reluctance to distress her parents by sharing her own pain, they ultimately provided the foundation for a healing experience for all the family members. Not surprisingly, the young woman was able to graduate from high school on time and in the following fall went on to college, where she once again was able to perform successfully.

PART II

Grief in the Context of Therapy

❧

CHAPTER 11

Creating Funerals, Ceremonies, and Other Healing Rituals

∾

"I'm pregnant," my daughter told me hesitantly, on the phone. She and her boyfriend hadn't known each other very long, and this baby was not planned. Quickly I realized how important my reaction in this moment would be for the future, and just as quickly I knew that I wanted to welcome this new life into our family, no matter what the circumstances. "That's wonderful," I said, "I'm so happy for you!" We lived 1,700 miles apart and hadn't seen each other more than twice a year for several years. It seemed that she "needed her space." Now I had an excuse to call her more often. I hoped that the pregnancy and the birth of her child would bring us closer together.

On Mother's Day she phoned me, her voice pained, saying she was unable to get comfortable in any position. "Are you in labor?" I asked. She moaned, "I can't be, I'm only 32 weeks." Very late that night the phone rang again. Her boyfriend left a message: "Your daughter is in labor." Instantly awake, I phoned the hospital. The baby would be born soon. I immediately arranged for a plane flight and started packing. Two hours later I got the call—TWINS! No one had known! When the boy was born, the midwife had said, "There's another baby in there!" And the little girl came 7 minutes later, just before the doctor arrived.

Because the babies were so small, they were taken immediately to a larger hospital for a higher level of care. I arrived that afternoon and saw my first grandchildren on the first day of their lives. For this grandma, just being present with their pure newborn energy was an honor and a privilege. Holding them in my arms was a thrill of a lifetime, blissful and deeply fulfilling.

I bought two baby books—one for the girl and one for the boy. I wanted to chronicle every new thing they did. These baby books were substantial: the large size, from birth to 5 years old. There were pages to fill with all the information you would ever want to know about the parents and grandparents, their gifts and visits. There were pages for the babies' firsts: first smile, first tooth, first step. There was even a page about the world into which they had just been born: popular songs, political leaders, sports figures. I felt proud to be fixing this moment in time for them, to give them a personal and family history of pride and caring.

The books quickly took on a life of their own as they became filled with memories of the babies' first days. Photographs of the babies with their mommy and daddy, grandparents, and uncle were added to the books as soon as they were developed. Soon, the little boy's book showed pictures of him going home from the hospital. He could lie on his tummy and push himself up with his arms, lifting up his head—already! The picture to prove it went into his baby book.

But his twin sister wasn't thriving. The second night of her life she needed surgery to alleviate an intestinal obstruction. Her parents and grandparents waited in the hospital until 2:30 in the morning, when the surgeon told us the painful news. The surgery was not successful. What is more, the doctors believed she had cystic fibrosis. Tests over the next few days confirmed the diagnosis.

We spent hours in the hospital with her—holding her, rocking her, watching her sleep. My daughter and I refused to believe that she wouldn't survive. After all, we were told, some people with cystic fibrosis live to be 30 years old. We kept a positive attitude. She was on prayer lists all over the country. We were open for a miracle.

The doctors tried many things to help unblock the obstruction. For a while, she seemed to improve. She was able to drink milk from the breast, to my daughter's great delight. But then, she wasn't able to digest the milk. The problem was still there.

On the 27th day of her life, she had another surgery. We stayed up all night, waiting, exhausted, until the surgeon emerged to tell us they were not able to repair our little girl's intestines, which were perforated in many places. It looked like there was no hope.

Still, we refused to give up. We prayed. I stood beside her for hours, holding her little hand, talking with her, telling her how much I loved her, visualizing all the fun we would have together singing and dancing and playing. I tried by sheer force of will to keep her with us. But it was not to be. Twenty-nine days after she was born, she died.

We were devastated.

Heartbroken, I privately took out all the future pages of the little girl's baby book. There would be no first tooth, no first step, no first word. Passionately and obsessively, I poured all my anguish, my feelings of helplessness, anger and failure, into the aching, bittersweet labor of detailing every special moment of our precious girl's life, in words and pictures, as if by capturing these moments, we could keep her with us. Her birth certificate, her hospital bracelet, her little comb, all proved that she had had a life, however brief. From my journal, I wrote a narrative, the story of her life. I wanted everyone to know that in that short life she had made a connection with all of us. She had touched me deeply, forever.

The day of her memorial service was painfully gorgeous. It had been raining for days, dark and gloomy, but suddenly this day was bright, sunny, and warm. Mount Rainier dazzled in the distance beyond the deep blue waters of the sound. How could it be so beautiful when our darling was gone?

At the graveside, we placed a heart-shaped wreath of pink and white flowers, and on either side of the wreath, two enlarged photographs—one, of my granddaughter looking up at her mommy and daddy with her little hand around Daddy's finger, and the other of my daughter holding her twins in her arms. Surrounding these were sprays of flowers sent by my parents, my brothers and sisters, and their families. Right in the center in front (at the heart of the display) I put the baby book.

People were drawn to the book, tenderly turning the pages, smiling and crying at the photographs of our girl looking up at her mommy or looking at her daddy. "It looks like she's smiling," they said. "She was so beautiful." "She looked like her mommy."

After the service, we gathered at the home of the other grandparents. People gathered around the book, reading all about this baby's parents and grandparents: where they went to school, where they lived, their favorite pastimes. We shared our caring, our pain, and our love through the story and the photographs in the book. We laughed through our tears. Focusing on the book helped to bring us all close, even people who had never met each other.

Two months later, at a family reunion on my side of the family, my daughter brought her daughter's baby book to share with the family members who never got to see her. One by one, they lingered over the book, with smiles and tears. The little girl's radiant spirit shone out to everyone, uniting us all in love and empathy.

Creating the baby book for my grandchildren was intensely powerful for me. For the child who died, I was completely absorbed in my intention to create a beautiful, meaningful celebration of her life, a testament to how much she was loved. I wanted to show how deeply she had touched me and how grateful I was for all that her presence had given me. Sharing the joy and heartbreak of her life and death also brought me much closer to my daughter and the baby's father, as well as to our new in-laws, as we bonded together to support our children.

Now when I look through the baby book, I savor every page; every photograph evokes a rich memory and feeling for me. Some of the images are unbearably sad; some are unspeakably lovely.

I didn't get to keep my first granddaughter, but her baby book keeps her sweet memory alive and real. Through this book, she will always be with us.

—KAL

Since time immemorial, socially sanctioned rituals, traditions, and ceremonies have been the vehicle for transmitting group beliefs and expectations as well as for maintaining order within a given culture. Worship services, weddings, funerals, rites of initiation, naming ceremonies, and holiday observances are some of the many forms rituals may take. In addition to supplying the standards for what is considered to be appropriate behavior in various circumstances, formal rituals also serve many functions. At a fundamental level, they sustain continuity with the past, offer stability in the present, and provide guidance for the future. The mechanism for this process has been described as follows:

> They transmit the combined wisdom of previous generations and are built on the promise that future generations can derive the lessons of painful experiences without having to repeat them. Rituals, like myths, address (1) our urge to comprehend our existence in a meaningful way, (2) our search for a marked pathway as we move from one stage of our lives to the next, (3) our need to establish secure and fulfilling relationships within a human community, and (4) our longing to know our part in the vast wonder and mystery of the cosmos. Rituals carry the mythology generated by the culture in response to these needs, and they translate that mythology into the individual's experience. (Feinstein, 1990, p. 41)

Rituals thus are basic to the structure of a society and to its well-being. And they also serve crucial roles at various other levels of the society. For example, rituals have been found to be significant contributors to the healthy functioning of families (Becvar, 1985; Imber-Black, 1991; Otto, 1979; Sawin, 1979, 1982; Wolin & Bennett, 1984). In a general sense, rituals have the potential to increase a sense of group identity within families. They also may create continuity at the same time that they allow for growth, change, and the accommodation of loss (Becvar & Becvar, 2000). Specifically, a different context often emerges for families through the creation and implementation of rituals and ceremonies. Indeed, in this regard it has been noted that "all family relationship systems seem to unlock during the months before and after such events, and it is often possible to open doors (or close them) between various family members with less effort during these intensive periods than could ordinarily be achieved with years of agonizing efforts" (Friedman, 1980, p. 430).

Rituals and ceremonies also may offer many benefits to the individual participants. With their emphasis on content as well as process, rituals tap into and acknowledge both tangible and intangible realities (Gunn, 1980). They also imply action and thus may transform feelings of powerless into a greater sense of control. Given their prescribed form and predictability, they have the power to "give shape to joy, form to grief, and order to the assertion of might—and in so doing contain and relieve our anxieties" (LaFarge, 1982, p. 64). In addition, rituals play an important role in the ability to release deeply felt emotions and feelings as a function of the way that we may respond to or be touched by them: "The purpose of ritual is to use symbolism that speaks to our souls. It connects with us at a spiritual level and gradually conditions us to enter light trance states upon the experience of the various stimuli present in the ritual" (Madden, 1999, p. 159).

Unfortunately, however, despite the importance attributed to rituals it is the conclusion of many social scientists that we live in a period characterized by "the erosion of ancient traditions" (Scanzoni, 1981, p. 796). What is more, the lack of meaningful traditions and ceremonies at a societal level is cited by some as a sign of decay within the culture (Feinstein, 1990). That is, we appear to be in grave danger of "losing the sense of historical continuity, the sense of belonging to a succession of generations originating in the past and stretching into the future" (Lasch, 1979, p. 30). As a result, there are those who believe that we as individuals, as families, and as a society may suffer serious consequences:

> It is probably one of the basic illnesses of modern time that in our left-hemispheric *hubris* we have banished ritual from our lives. For while we apparently succeeded in performing this excision, the age-old longing for the mystery of rituals remains unfulfilled and either contributes to an acute feeling of senselessness and emptiness, or attaches itself to such pitiful substitutes as the acquisition of a driver's license instead of a rite of initiation. (Watzlawick, 1978, p. 155)

In addition to an absence relative to meaningful rites of initiation for young people, certainly the realm of death and dying is an area in which a diminishing respect for rituals and traditions also may be observed. As one writer notes, "We live in a time when people have a lot of negative attitudes about funeral rituals. Some dismiss them as archaic!" (Smith, 1996, p. 51). Further, although there also are many others who do not find funerals archaic, some may choose to avoid them because of negative experiences in the past. As mentioned in Chapter 1, even when traditional funeral rites are observed they may feel like empty exercises given the lack of involvement and personalization on the part of those most closely related to the deceased.

Nevertheless, we might do well to recognize that rituals have the potential to play a vital role not only in our ability to function well in the good times but also in our efforts to cope successfully in the bad times. Funerals, ceremonies, and other healing rituals provide opportunities to honor and recognize the person who has died. They also offer a context for social support and emotional release for those who are bereaved. What is more, whether through revising old traditions or creating new ones, family members may be assisted in the process of coming to terms with the death and learning to create a new life in the absence of a loved one.

The discussions in this chapter therefore focus, in turn, on each of the following three areas: Beginning with the process of designing funerals, I consider both the benefits to be derived from carefully created rites and the freedom we as individuals may have to be full and active participants from the moment of death until the ritual is completed. Included in the latter regard is an examination of both traditional and nontraditional options. I then turn to the steps involved with planning various kinds of ceremonies related to the death of a loved one. Such ceremonies may provide a way to fill a void created when a funeral was not held previously. They may offer a way to redo services considered in retrospect to have been unsatisfactory. And they may supplement funerals and add a sense of completion when that is what seems appropriate. Finally, I describe the process of developing other healing rituals. Included in this section is a review of a variety of ways to help those who are bereaved get through the holidays successfully, ideas for marking the anniversary of a death, and suggestions both for memorializing the person who has died and for supporting those who survive.

DESIGNING FUNERALS

Funerals, like rituals and traditions in general, serve a multitude of functions that extend far beyond the most obvious purpose of bidding farewell in the context of a particular set of religious or spiritual beliefs. Such services acknowledge the loss and pain of the survivors, allowing for the open expression of grief (Imber-Black, 1991). They also offer an opportunity for public recognition of the death (Kastenbaum, 1986) as well as affirmation of the life of the person who has died. They provide as well a setting in which to consider and speak about the meaning of both death and life.

In addition, funerals serve the public purpose of disposing appropriately of the body (Kastenbaum, 1986). In some religious traditions they also support the process of transition for the deceased while providing comfort for the survivors (Starhawk & The Reclaiming Collective, 1997). And whether spiritual or secular, they create a context that facilitates connection with a community of support (Imber-Black, 1991). Indeed, a funeral may be thought of as "a formalized gathering time and place for friends as well as for family to grieve. The gatherings can become something of a reunion, especially when conversations begin, " 'Do you remember the time . . .' " (Smith, 1996, p. 51).

Thus, although family members may be reluctant to deal in more than a superficial way, or even at all, with the myriad of details involved with planning a funeral, as helpers we might encourage them to think carefully before making a decision in this regard. In addition to pointing out the potential benefits of a carefully planned and executed funeral, we also might help to allay some of the common fears these family members are experiencing. For example, they may be familiar with stories about the exorbitant costs involved with embalming and the purchase of a coffin; indeed, for quite some time the funeral industry has been under serious scrutiny relative to such concerns and many of these fears are not unwarranted (Mitford, 1963, 2000).

Those who are bereaved also may have attended other funerals they believe did not truly honor or do justice either to the person who died or to his or her family. They thus may be worried about the lack of control they believe they are likely to have over what ultimately transpires. They also may be intimidated by those whom they perceive to be in positions of authority. However, despite the pressure survivors may feel, funeral directors are there to carry out the wishes of those who are purchasing their services (Kastenbaum, 1986). Moreover, there are many ways to keep the costs manageable and if the person is clear about his or her wishes, they can be met. Similarly, the bereaved person does not necessarily have to abide by all the rules prescribed by a particular religious tradition.

For example, when my son died, I knew immediately that I wanted little to do with a funeral home. I did not like the heavy, formal feeling that such places usually exude and knew that it just would not be appropriate given the circumstances. Because of the cause of death and the damage to my son's body, we opted for cremation. And because an autopsy was required by law in Missouri in the case of accidental death, we also had to accept the fact that there might be a delay in the proceedings. I met first with our Episcopal priest, telling him that I wanted whatever services there would be to be held at the church. We planned a vigil for one evening and a memorial mass for the following morning. I selected the hymns and some favorite poems, designed the program to be distributed to those who attended and informed him that there were four people who I would like to have speak. (It was only much later that I learned that Episcopalians do not typically permit outside speakers to participate in the service!)

Accompanied by my husband, my daughter, my children's father, and the priest, we met for several hours with the funeral directors. This was my one and only visit to the funeral home. There, we handled all the paper work, prepared the obituary notice for the newspaper, selected the coffin for the cremation, and agreed that the funeral home would do the transporting to and from the crematorium. Although the timing was tight, the ashes arrived in time for the evening vigil and were placed on the altar in a small side chapel. The church was filled to overflowing and I believe that both services were beautiful and meaningful tributes to my son.

At the time, which was in late August, we did not have a cemetery plot. I therefore chose to leave the ashes at the church, where they remained for several months. When I finally was able to search out and locate the appropriate spot in a small cemetery, I planned a private committal service. All this was transpiring as I traveled back and forth between Texas and Missouri. We also had to wait until Christmas break, when all our family members would be together.

I purchased a permanent container for the ashes through another funeral home nearer our church. The priest offered to bring the ashes, placed in the container, to the cemetery on the day in January selected for the service. My husband and several friends dug the grave, the priest performed a brief service, and a few of us shared prayers from various religious traditions. We then had a small gathering at our home. In the months that followed, I designed and had a stone cut to mark my son's grave. And when spring came, and the ground had warmed and softened, my husband and I went back and placed the stone in the ground ourselves.

Although it may be difficult to go against the norm or change the rules, it is often worth the effort. Moreover, this is where others less closely related may provide a real service. First of all, the survivors need to be helped to decide what type of arrangements *they* desire and how *they* would like things to be handled. Then they would benefit greatly from moral support as they go through the process of meeting with funeral directors and clergy persons. And, finally, they need affirmation that what they are doing is in the best interests of those who survive and supports as well the wishes of the person who has died.

Helpers also may provide additional information about the variety of options available relative to caring for the body of the deceased and preparation for burial or cremation. For example, it is legal in most states for family members to care for their own dead (Carlson, 1987; Kreilkamp, 1999). Indeed, in many states all arrangements for funerals, end-of-life documentation, and transportation of the deceased may be handled by a family member or a person with a Durable Power of Attorney for Health Care. If one chooses to create a home ceremony, it may be important to know that dry ice will sustain the body for 3 days, thereby removing the necessity for embalming. It also is possible to purchase, for less than $35, plans to build either a wooden casket for burial or a cardboard casket for cremation.

In terms of the funeral service, there are certainly many options. The problem is that in the midst of great grief it is sometimes hard to remember that one has choice. Therefore, we may help family members by listening sensitively, carefully exploring possibilities, and encouraging them to trust their intuitive sense, their feelings about what seems right. We also may make thoughtful suggestions and offer ideas and information based on experience with others. For example, the idea of celebrating the life of the person who has died in addition to mourning his or her death may prove to be comforting. Choosing those who will participate as pallbearers also may be important. To illustrate, I recently attended a funeral in which the coffin of the deceased was attended by the members of the band in which the son was a member. This choice had been made because attending the band's performances had been such an important and enjoyable experience for the father.

There also are many people who desire to be cremated and to have their ashes scattered in a place that was meaningful to them during their lifetime. In such instances, it may be useful to discuss the importance of creating a ritual to accompany the dispersal of the ashes. At the same time it also is important to be aware that after the ashes are scattered, however appropriately handled, survivors may be troubled by the fact that there is no cemetery or grave site to visit. For this and a variety of other reasons, it also may be useful to think about creating special ceremonies.

PLANNING CEREMONIES

Ceremonies may be small or large, public or private, and they may be planned to achieve any number of goals. For example, if survivors who have followed the wishes of the deceased to be cremated and to have the ashes scattered also desire to create a specific place that honors their loved one, they may choose to simply plant a tree as a memorial or they may wish to create a more elaborate shrine. In the latter case, they may wish to have a plaque inscribed with the name and dates of the deceased and to place it in the midst of flowers and shrubs, and perhaps a pond or fountain. They may wish to have a small bench placed there so that they may use the spot as a place to pray or just sit. Whether or not they choose to invite others to participate in the planting of the tree or the blessing of the shrine is strictly a matter of personal preference. What may be most important is that they find a way to add closure at the same time that they create a place that provides a focus for their grief.

Closure may be an even more significant issue if no ceremony was held at the time of the death. This is often the case when a miscarriage occurs or a baby dies (Khoner & Henley, 1997). Perhaps the hospital handled all the arrangements. Perhaps the parents were too upset at the time to think about a funeral. Perhaps they do not even know what happened to their baby's body. Although the reasons for such circumstances may have made sense at the time, in subsequent years they may have become the cause of great distress for bereaved parents: "Many have a feeling of 'unfinished business'. They feel that they should have marked their baby's life and death in some way and made a proper ending to their experience. Not having done so, they find they can neither grieve as they want to grieve, nor allow their grief to rest" (Khoner & Henley, 1997, p. 89).

Regardless of the number of years that have passed as well as whether or not the baby's body is able to be located, it is possible to plan a ceremony that allows the family to make a more formal farewell and thereby to find some comfort and peace. At such a ceremony they may express the hopes and dreams they had during the pregnancy. They may talk about the sadness they feel about only having been able to have the child be a part of their lives for a short time. Including traditional prayers or music may be a source of comfort. Inviting significant others and choosing an appropriate place for the ceremony also may lend important dimensions. What is most crucial is that such a ceremony may help to fill in the void that was created not only by the baby's death but also by the previous lack of a formal ritual.

There also are times, even when a funeral or other ritual has been held, when some of the participants may feel that something additional is needed. Perhaps a group of friends may wish to create a ceremony that speaks specifically to their own needs and honors one or more of their number who has died. Thus, they may wish to plan a public ritual, for example, "the Naming of Names" (Smith, 1996, p. 158), in which friends gather and participate in a formal ceremony that addresses their losses and speaks to their friendships. Conversely, when one member of a group of close friends has died, the other members may wish to do something that is a strictly private way of paying their respects to the deceased.

In either case, they might include a candlelighting ceremony. Each person who attends might be invited to share a favorite anecdote as well as offer a poem, a prayer, or other reading in memory of a specific friend. They might prepare and share food together or laugh and cry together. The goal of such ceremonies is to provide a context which allows friends to express their grief, support each other, and bid farewell in their own unique ways to the person who has died.

The following anecdote describes a memorial service which was created for just such reasons. In this case, however, the ceremony included friends, coworkers, and family members. The central figure is Mimi, a beloved mother, grandmother, and friend to many:

> When Mimi died, only the immediate family attended the graveside funeral service, in accordance with her wishes. But so many people wanted to pay their respects to this wonderful woman that Ron [her son] organized a memorial service at home the day after the funeral. For nearly two hours (captured on video), more than one hundred friends, family members, and coworkers shared their memories of this beloved woman. They extolled a woman who saw only the good in everyone, who was a great sport, willing to try new experiences, passionately devoted to her family, and who made the world's best chicken soup. It was an extraordinary outpouring, marked with tears, laughter, and the love that was Mimi's legacy. (Brooks, 1999, p. 59)

Ceremonies thus may supplement, they may fill a void, or they may complement. Moreover, in addition to meeting needs where family members and friends are concerned, a simple ceremony in honor of a beloved animal who has died also may be helpful for bereaved pet owners. However, although as adults we may give ourselves permission to create a ritual for the benefit of children when an animal dies, we may be reluctant to do something similar for ourselves. We may feel it is foolish or inappropriate. Nevertheless, there is nothing wrong with acknowledging an important loss, regardless of our age. And, as discussed in the previous chapter, the death of a pet can be mourned as deeply as the loss of the relationship with another human. Thus, as helpers our endorsement of a ceremony may prove beneficial. Similarly, we may provide ideas regarding how to conduct such a ceremony.

As we assist family members and friends in planning ceremonies, several important factors should be considered (Becvar, 1985). First, we would do well to discuss with those involved what it is they hope to accomplish. A focus on their goals will help to guide the creation of the format as well as the planning of other critical details. As we become clear about what it is they desire, we also may be able to help keep their expectations within reasonable limits.

Second, we may be able to assist them in maintaining an emphasis on the positive, on the growth-producing aspects of the situation as well as on the strengths of everyone involved. Thus, for example, they may be encouraged to include humor as well as seriousness, particularly if this fits with the person who died. And as they negotiate the details of the arrangements, particularly if there is disagreement or conflict, we may be able to help them to keep in mind their intent to honor the deceased and what her or his wishes might have been relative to the issues at hand.

Third, we may suggest either the inclusion or exclusion of others, depending on the circumstances. That is, it may seem overwhelming for some to have to express private thoughts and feelings in a public way. Some also may not want to have to worry about having too many around or be concerned with the idea of having to "entertain" additional people. By contrast, for some the presence of others outside the immediate family may feel supportive. Indeed, the absence of others might be perceived as diminishing the meaningfulness of the ceremony.

Fourth, as part of the planning we might remind family members and friends of the importance of affirmation for the survivors as well as for the deceased. In other words, it may be appropriate that the ceremony be planned to recognize the meaning of the loss for the living as well to memorialize the one who has died. It thus may be useful to incorporate into the occasion a sense of its sacredness as well as an attitude of celebration.

Finally, though it is necessary to keep factors such as the foregoing in mind, we also must remember that our primary role is that of consultant rather than creator. Indeed, a crucial part of the power of a ritual derives from the process of designing and bringing it into being. As family members or friends work together to plan the ceremony it becomes uniquely their own. And the more they feel a sense of ownership, the more likely it is that the ceremony will be supportive of their healing. Similarly, just as all these considerations are important to keep in mind when planning ceremonies, they also are worthy of attention as we work with others to develop additional healing rituals that will support their ability to continue living and to function well in the presence of grief.

DEVELOPING RITUALS

Certainly another avenue by means of which we may offer assistance with the process of living after loss is the sharing of ideas about rituals and the creation or re-creation of personal and family traditions. Indeed, everyday life may be understood as a series of rituals, for example, relative to ways of getting up in the morning, fixing and eating meals, and preparing for bed, as well as a variety of other regular, daily routines. All these rituals and routines are likely to be interrupted or at least disturbed by the death of a loved one, thereby increasing the sense of dislocation experienced by those who are grieving. However, by recognizing their importance and the need for a specific focus that enables change in this area, we may be able to provide invaluable support. What is more, whether large or small, one is limited only by imagination in the potential to develop meaningful and healing rituals.

For example, initially it may be important for a husband or wife whose spouse has died to keep their house, and particularly their bedroom, just as it was. This may be a source of stability that enables the survivor to begin to assimilate his or her loss. Over time, however, it may become more appropriate to begin to think about rearranging furniture and shifting the organization of the household. Such changes symbolically acknowledge and mark the alteration in the structure of life occasioned by the death.

There are also many other opportunities for the development of healing rituals relative to the challenge of dealing with daily living. A major issue may involve figuring out what to do with the room of a child or other family member. For some, it may be most helpful to dispose of the belongings of the person who has died and to change the purpose for which the room is used. For others, it may be more appropriate to keep things just as they were in an attempt to create a kind of memorial, or a place to which to retreat. In the latter case, taking time on a daily basis to sit in the room and think about the loved one, just being quiet, or perhaps meditating or praying, may allow an individual to get through the rest of the day in a more peaceful manner.

A related ritual, one that may be especially meaningful during the early phases of mourning, is to spend time on a regular basis writing in a journal. Such a journal provides an opportunity to note what is happening as the individual struggles through each day. It also provides a repository for a variety of thoughts and feelings. Sometimes, just having the opportunity to get painful emotions "off one's chest" may help to lighten the burden of grief. And, in retrospect, having such a record enables the survivor to look back and understand the distance she or he has traveled on the journey to healing.

Similarly, a person may be encouraged to plan a regular time and space in which to be alone for the purpose of focusing on his or her grief. During this alone time, the bereaved person may hold something that belonged to the deceased. This may be a time to speak to the person who has died, either aloud or in one's mind. This also may be a time just to listen. By allowing a time to cry as well as to communicate, a feeling of control over the grief may be fostered even as a sense of continuing connection with the loved one may be fostered.

When just getting dressed in the morning seems like too much effort, perhaps the bereaved person can be encouraged to wear an article of clothing, such as a shirt, that belonged to the person who died. One woman also had necklaces made for herself and her daughters from medals that had belonged to her husband. Another woman continues to wear only the earrings that were a gift to her from her daughter at the last birthday they celebrated together before the daughter's death. Each time they put on the article of clothing or the jewelry they feel a sense of closeness as well as a reminder of special times they spent together with the one who died.

In addition to daily routines, dealing with holidays also tends to be challenging following the death of a family member. In the words of the father of five whose youngest son had died in a mountain climbing accident: "The worst days now are holidays: Thanksgiving, Easter, Pentecost, birthdays, weddings, January 31—days meant as festivals of happiness and joy are now days of tears. The gap is too great between day and heart. Days of routine I can manage; no songs are expected. But how am I to sing in this desolate land, when there's always one too few" (Wolterstorff, 1987, p. 61).

Indeed, those most closely related to the deceased person may feel overwhelmed and may be reluctant even to observe the holiday. What is more, should they decide to proceed, all those who ultimately participate may not know whether to speak or to be silent about the person who has died. In cases in which conversation would be considered appropriate and welcome, a place for the person who died may be set at the family dinner table. This may decrease the uncertainty and allow for greater comfort as the absence is openly acknowledged and feelings, memories, and other thoughts are encouraged and shared openly. It is in the context of such occasions that the loved one's absence is often most apparent. Thus, paying explicit attention to this reality may prove helpful, particularly to the bereaved.

Birthdays of the deceased as well as the anniversary of her or his death also may be anticipated with dread. However, if the bereaved person is able to create a regular routine by means of which to get through these days, their meaning may shift in a more welcoming direction. Accordingly, these may be the days designated for a visit to the cemetery and/or participation in an activity or taking a trip to a place that was preferred by the person who died. Such days also may include cooking and eating his or her best loved foods or going to his or her favorite restaurant. The bereaved person may want to choose particular people with whom to share such events on an annual basis. The birthdays and anniversaries thereby may take on the dual meaning of remembering the person who died and demonstrating gratitude for the support of others.

When a birthday or holiday that involves gift giving comes around, other options also are available. Perhaps the amount of money that previously would have been used to purchase gifts for the person who died may be donated to someone of comparable age. Perhaps the survivor might buy the gifts and deliver them to a social service agency with an outreach to those less fortunate and where they would be greatly appreciated. Perhaps the bereaved might think about "adopting" a family in need in order to help them through the holidays by providing food and gifts. Each of these options could be exercised in memory of the person who died and also might help those who survive to feel better about the holiday.

In addition, regardless of the occasion, the lighting of a memorial candle may offer a sense of the loved one's presence, in this instance without the need for words. Indeed, such a candle may be unobtrusive and perhaps out of the awareness of anyone other than those who choose to light it. Nevertheless, it may provide a gentle and silent reminder of the fact that no matter how many times the occasion previously has been celebrated, it can never again be experienced in the same old way, nor is the missing person forgotten. When the lighting of the candle is accompanied by a prayer or blessing, it also offers an additional way to honor the memory of the person who has died.

An activity that may be particularly helpful, and one that can be pursued slowly in the weeks and months following a death, is to create a scrapbook, photograph album, or some other type of collection. The goal may be to capture the highlights of the life of the person who died or simply to recapture a special event. For example, a client whose husband had died 5 years previously spent many months redoing and creating annotations for the pictures in her wedding album. Activities such as this certainly may elicit tears, but they also are likely to evoke many happy memories which may become the basis for support and healing. In addition, they may offer an opportunity to invite participation by others. In either case,

> It is better for us to help our memories live. We can do this by recording on tape, or in writing, the things our loved one said, the way he or she looked or acted. We may record our special moments, the times we most enjoyed together. We may assemble notes, photographs, letters, and clippings in one central place so that we will have a tangible memory bank that we can visit any time we wish. We can also invite others who know our loved one to contribute their special memories and observations. (Smith, 1996, p. 130)

Other healing rituals also may be appropriate, for example, to mend relationships characterized by conflict or to provide closure to unfinished business. Writing letters to the deceased and then perhaps reading aloud what was written may enable survivors to feel that they can release old issues or at least decrease their potency. Such activities may be concluded by burning the letter or letters, thereby further symbolizing the process of letting go.

Finding ways to volunteer or do for others in a manner the bereaved person feels she or he did not do adequately for the person who died also may be helpful in alleviating guilt feelings. For example, perhaps a daughter or son was unable because of distance to spend a great deal of time with a dying parent. Such a person might be encouraged to become a visitor at a retirement center or nursing home. If working with the elderly is not a comfortable choice, she or he might think about volunteering in a hospital or community center for children.

Becoming involved in a cause, particularly when a sense of injustice surrounds the death, has the potential to help with the process of regaining a measure of equanimity. Indeed, many well-known bereavement groups were created by survivors as part of an attempt to prevent what happened to them from happening to others. By doing so, the founders of groups such as Mothers Against Drunk Drivers and Parents of Murdered Children also found a way to direct their grief and anger into productive channels.

Though few of us may have the energy or inclination to create or participate regularly in groups such as these, many do offer rituals that may be helpful on a time-limited or a one-time-only basis. For example, the Compassionate Friends, a national support group for the parents, and in some cases the siblings, of children who have died hosts a candle-lighting ceremony in our area each year at the holiday season. Similarly, hospitals often sponsor support groups and periodically hold special services to remember those who have died. The important issue to keep in mind is a choice of activity that fits with the needs of the bereaved person and alleviates rather than enhances his or her grief.

Indeed, as with every other aspect of the grieving process, creating funerals, ceremonies, and other healing rituals is a personal process. As helpers, we provide the greatest service by sharing ideas, providing information, and supporting realistic choices. And, in each case, the hope is that we also may support what is perhaps the most important task and most difficult challenge when living or working in the presence of grief—the search for meaning.

THERAPEUTIC CONVERSATIONS AND REFLECTIONS

∾

I had been working for several months with a middle-age woman whose child, the third of five, had been killed in an automobile accident 2 years previously. She had come to therapy seeking assistance with the process of regaining a sense of equilibrium for herself and her family. I had met with the entire family periodically and agreed with my client's perception that, all things considered, things seemed to be proceeding rather well.

Just prior to the Christmas holidays, however, my client came in reporting deep distress. Apparently her children, who ranged in age from 12 to 20, had informed her that they wanted to cancel

(cont.)

Christmas. The two older children were the ringleaders, but the two younger ones were going along. The parents were in a quandary regarding how to respond and were looking for suggestions I might have to help them with their answer.

My client acknowledged that the first Christmas after her child's death had been extremely painful. However, she believed that they had managed to limp through it fairly well and even to have some fun. For that holiday the parents had invited some close friends to be with them and this seemed to have helped somewhat in dealing with their changed circumstances. By the second Christmas, however, they decided to celebrate alone. Unfortunately, the obvious void left by the child who died seemed to cast a pall over everything. Mom was aware that her children continued to have difficulty with most holidays. Nevertheless she was surprised at the depth of their feelings about Christmas.

As far as Christmas was concerned, it was important for the parents to try to re-create some of the joy they had experienced with previous celebrations. This was a holiday that had great significance for both religious and secular reasons, having always been one of the most meaningful and happiest of family events. The parents felt that if they were to accede to their children's wishes they ultimately would do them and the family a great disservice. Their desire was to focus on creating new, happy memories for themselves as well as for their children despite the tragedy they had experienced.

As we talked, I learned that since their child's death, the parents had attempted to maintain to the fullest extent possible all their old rituals, continuing to celebrate Christmas as they always had. Their tradition was that the family went to church together on Christmas eve. On Christmas morning they had breakfast and then Mom got the turkey in the oven. Next followed the ritual of gift giving. Packages, which had been placed under the tree, were distributed and opened by each person in turn until no more remained. Given the size of the family this process took several hours and was concluded with the opening of Christmas stockings. The family would then relax and "hang out" until dinner was served. After dinner and cleanup, they watched a movie together.

After discussing the fact that part of the dilemma the children were experiencing might have something to do with the attempt to keep things as they always had been, I suggested that the parents put their heads together and consider how they could still have Christmas this year but do it differently. My client agreed to discuss this with her husband and eventually they devised a whole new scenario. They then convened a family meeting at which time they read a letter inviting the family to consider doing things in a new way.

The plan called for the family to open gifts on Christmas eve. Rather than placing gifts under the tree, each person's packages would be in separate spots around the house. The family would move as a group from one "station" to the next, and at each station the appropriate person would open one of her or his gifts. They would save the stockings for the next day, however. In the morning, the family would have breakfast and then go to church together. When they got home, they would open their stocking gifts. Friends would be invited to dinner to be held in mid-afternoon. After dinner they would all sing some carols and/or play games together. The letter was signed, "Santa Claus."

The children agreed to give the plan a try and Mom reported after the holidays that things had gone surprisingly well. It remains to be seen, of course, how the family rituals will evolve over time. In fact, at some point they may shift back to be more consistent with the earlier tradition. However, at the moment the radical changes coupled with the parents' willingness to be flexible seem to have enabled the family to prevent a crisis and to move successfully through a difficult time.

In reflecting on these events, it seems important to emphasize that the particular holiday is not what is truly significant. Indeed, the same issues might arise around Hanukkah, or Kwaanza or a holiday unrelated to any religious or spiritual tradition. What we most need to recognize is that memories are embedded in rituals. As old routines are reenacted, they inevitably call to mind what happened in the past as well as the way things "should be" now. Thus, a person's absence becomes even more apparent and the ritual becomes painful as what once was a source of stability is now a reminder of the degree to which things have changed. Stability and change require each other in an ongoing balancing act in which the focus shifts alternately from one end of the continuum to the other. In this instance, to remain stable, it was necessary for the family to accept and accommodate change.

CHAPTER 12

Searching for Meaning

∿

October 24, 1998

She was my big sister, 4 years my senior. I guess, as kids, I thought she was bossy. As adolescents, she was always busy, always on the go, involved in committees of sorts, extracurricular classes and crafts, heading some cause or another, leading such an active social life that she sometimes challenged our father's conservative household rules. She left for college in St. Louis when I was in my early teens and we didn't spend meaningful time together again until we were both adults. She was still my big sister though, and would cheer me on from afar when I encountered success, letting me know, as well, when she saw things differently than I did, still supporting me in the process—as a big sister would.

So, I guess I always knew that she was what I would call a "No Nonsense Lady." But it was only in the recent years, gradually, through our occasional visits and in seeing her through the eyes of other people who lived and worked closely with her on a day-to-day basis, that I came to understand that she was also an exceptional human being.

I know now that my sister, in her simplicity, led an extraordinary life, a life of attending quickly, efficiently, and unassumingly to the business at hand, whether it be cooking, teaching, sewing, writing, or learning to befriend her cancer. In activities that were important to her, the pursuit of excellence was a given. She frequently found the appropriate spices and garnishes to convert a simple meal into a gourmet event. She corrected her nieces' and nephews' grammar and punctuation—as well as that of us adults around her when she couldn't help herself. But she also included snippets of their work as well as stories about their learning in the books she wrote—pretty cool stuff when you're a kid to be included in a publication. Though probably she could have defeated me hands down at lots of word games, it was Boggle that she would ask to play when we were together, knowing full well that it was the one at which I would usually beat her. She enjoyed seeing people take pleasure in life and in learning, often taking a back seat as a quiet influence in making success happen.

She enriched her colleagues in their work and in their lives, gently coaching through questions, nudging, with smiles of encouragement, patience, and sometimes, most powerfully, with silence. She was a gracious and thoughtful hostess to her guests and a faithful correspondent to her friends, even from her hospital bed. She made sure that her visitors were all well-fed, often by the dishes that she had prepared for us ahead of time, while feeling ill, before her anticipated date of hospitalization. And she insisted that we go do our share of sightseeing in Seattle, unwilling to allow us to simply visit with her. She wrote her last thank-you notes to out-of-town guests on the day before they were to leave, which turned out to be her last as we knew her, in consciousness. But she had also begun to more easily allow others to care for her and love her, a lesson in vulnerability with which she felt her illness had challenged her.

My sister had continuously commanded her weakened body, even after her treatments, to perform, to exercise, and to eat in ways that most of us wouldn't even have contemplated under her circumstances, pushing forward toward her clearly set goals with commitment. Pain, discomfort, exhaustion, or tubes attached had often been irrelevant—she did what needed to be done, always taking the next steps with courage and persistence, never once complaining about her fate, and increasingly inspiring those of us who were privileged to witness her journey in search of healing. This journey, I gradually understood, was only a metaphor of what her life had been, as was the magnificent Mount Rainier that we were able to admire together, on clear days, from her hospital window. Her hope was to return, in health, to her life of teaching, mentoring, writing, and editing; to the new home which she loved; and to live to see more of the children in her world graduate from college. But she was grateful for the full, good life she had lived and seemed to have neither regrets nor fear about moving on, should moving on be what was in store.

And at the end of her quietly extraordinary living came an extraordinary dying, a tribute to who my sister was. She was surrounded by sweet and soothing sounds: of blessings, prayers shared and prayers silent, a tape of chanting that had comforted her in days past, "Amazing Grace" being sung to her, the sounds of loving messages of good-bye delivered to her, messages of gratitude, and wishes for serenity and peace from family, friends, colleagues, students, and caregivers. She was reminded of the first words of the American Indian poem that she had chosen to read at our mother's funeral, words that read, "Today is a good day to die. . . . " And then there were the sounds of her own breathing as it slowed, then slowed again, peacefully, gradually, until imperceptibly, she slipped away and breathed no more.

She died being touched tenderly, her soft, balded head being stroked and each hand being held gently, receiving total and unconditional love. She died with dignity and grace, as she had lived, her journey of healing completed.

October 10, 2000

It is wonderful what God can do with the broken heart, if He gets all the pieces.

> *The crucible for silver and the furnace for gold, but the Lord tests the heart.*
>
> Proverbs 17:3

I was given these words before my last trip to Seattle to be with my sister at the Hutchinson Cancer Research Center, weeks before her final health crisis was even anticipated. She was doing well in her recovery, our stem-cell transplant having successfully "taken." At the time I received this message, I read the words and they sounded beautiful. Today, two years later, I read them and they still sound beautiful—but they also resonate as truth.

When my mother died 3 years earlier, I had felt my heart truly was broken. Her death was a clear watershed for me, with befores and afters tinted by such a powerful period of transition, a transition that marked my soul as only a most meaningful rite of passage can. This, I understand now. Then, I could only experience the sometimes exquisite pain, wondering how one was to live with such sadness, how one was to move on, how people did move on. But I had found comfort on that first day, of death announced, in the love and compassion of shared sorrow, in the soothing and presence of those who cared for me, and in the reminders of a belief system that was challenged yet remained true. These sustained me through the day of the funeral and the day after, and the next day became 10, and then 10 more. I grieved without shame, without time frames, but with the patience and understanding of those who witnessed or shared in this process with me.

Yet, even in the midst of the existential confusion in which I was immersed, I knew that the pain was one of growth, of learning bittersweet but essential lessons, of glimpsing, in awe, God's wisdom in planning for darker threads in the outline of the salient features of a magnificent tapestry. I knew even then that the new threads woven were not in vain or accidental, and that the weaving would not cease. What I didn't know is how these seemingly dark threads would continue to mark my own life. At that time, I didn't foresee how our shared loss would bring us together differently as a family and prepare us to gather again around my sister's diagnosis of cancer, her journey thereafter, her eventual *death. As individuals and as family, we uncovered new fragility, we discovered new strengths.*

When my sister died, then, my sorrow was different. It was the sorrow of a sibling who had shared life and its sorrow and its hope and joy with her sister— no longer older or younger. It was more quiet and knowing. It was a bit more experienced, even a tiny bit wise. It knew about the tremendous gifts of ritual, and comfort, and healing. It understood that the end of a chapter had arrived, with the sadness of closing a great book, but with the knowledge and immense gratitude that the ending seemed to have been good. It recognized the pain re- membered, like the mother who experiences labor for a second time, sensing its sweetness too.

Still, I was surprised to gradually realize that this grief, while no less power- ful a rite of passage, was shaded in colors of softness, as soft as her bald head was when her wig no longer covered it. The memories that have invaded me over time—often unexpectedly as, in bereavement, memories do—have been sometimes unremarkable, sometimes striking, but all surprisingly comforting: Having a simple dinner of fresh salmon, salad and new red potatoes together at her new "home" in Seattle as she awaited her transplant, somehow treasuring the moment, with gratitude. The celebration of her "new birthday" on the day of the transplant. Walking into her hospital room after she became unconscious to find her peacefully sleeping, though hooked up to so much medical equipment— yet, in a bizarre way, looking so unpretentiously pretty to me. The precious inti- macy and vulnerability and humanity of the moment of her death. The final ferry ride we took in her honor and paid for with the last dollars from her purse before leaving Seattle. The walk to the funeral home, having collected along the way precious and simple symbols of all she had loved, of all who'd loved her, to be cremated in a little gift bag along with her body. Bittersweet memories, soft and caressing, broken pieces coming together moment by moment, one at a time.

The heart remains tender where it was wounded.
Yet, its healing becomes a great gift of love, a gift of ongoing life.

—DCC

The search to understand the meaning and significance of life, as well as to identify one's purpose while here, is rarely an easy process or one that is undertaken without some trepidation. However, when it is triggered by, or its importance is increased as a result of, the death of a loved one, such an undertaking is likely to be doubly daunting. If suddenly everything seems pointless, how can we hope to regain a sense of life as making sense? How can we ever imagine understanding and accepting a seemingly meaningless event? How can we begin to reconcile what we believed with what has happened? And yet, if ultimately we are to survive the loss well, to more than endure, this is exactly what we must attempt to do. Indeed, as noted by one researcher in the realm of loss, "The last and most difficult step in resolving any loss is to make sense of it" (Boss, 1999, p. 118).

However, as important as it thus may be for the bereaved to think about, and as challenging as it may be to begin to involve themselves in the process of searching for meaning, they also are faced with several additional dimensions of the dilemma. The first, and perhaps most discouraging, is the fact that where death is concerned there always will be more questions than there are answers. That is: "Death is one event that occurs in every society everywhere in the world, perhaps in the universe. And every society has a way of explaining death, each one believing that its way is the right way. Yet, I believe the truth remains that death is one event that our scientists know no more about than the sorcerers in New Guinea. We may know more about how dying occurs, at least the biological aspects, but none of use knows what death is" (Kalish, 1980, p. 2). What is more, although apparently we human beings are the only species who are aware of and thus can contemplate the awareness of our own death, we *cannot* know what it is or will be for each of us as long as we are alive.

In other words, it certainly is possible for individuals ultimately to attain new understanding and thereby to regain a feeling of stability even when their most cherished beliefs have been challenged or even destroyed. In a general sense, this may occur through the rewriting of old stories or the creation of new stories that serve us better in the context of changed circumstances. Nevertheless, they remain just that—useful stories. To explain, as with any theory about that which is intangible, we cannot know that what we believe to be true is indeed a true explanation. We, as the creators of our theories, or stories, cannot get outside of them, cannot have a "God's eye view" (Bronowski, 1978) by means of which to judge their truth or falseness in any absolute sense. Although we can acquire once again a sense that life is meaningful, at the same time, as one writer notes, "The question of meaning may linger indefinitely, however." (Kastenbaum, 1986, p. 144).

Accordingly, those who are bereaved are likely to find themselves engaged in a quest that could have several equally efficacious endings and yet may never end. As with life, it is thus the journey rather than the destination that becomes most significant. What is even more important to recognize is that the search for meaning is a process that is unique for each person, one that may unfold in many different directions. And probably the worst thing we can do is to try to force someone to travel a road that does not feel comfortable to that person. We therefore might do well to heed the words of one bereaved father: "My probing for meaning, I discover, is something very personal. I do not want a professional theologian to tell me how to interpret Dave's [my son's] death. I do not want other people to press their explanations on me. I react when a writer espouses a certain position as though any other is theologically naive or untenable" (Strommen & Strommen, 1993, p. 19).

It follows, then, that rather than attempting to provide answers, our goal must be to present ideas about how to encourage and support, in the most helpful way, the process of asking questions and of searching for meaning that is personally relevant. To provide assistance in this regard, this chapter begins with a discussion of further dimensions of the dilemma faced by bereaved persons relative to specific kinds of loss—parents who have lost a child, siblings who have lost a sister or brother, children who have lost their parents, wives or husbands who have lost a spouse, those who have lost a friend. In this discussion, I focus on the search for answers related to the larger meaning system that may have been undermined by the death as well as on questions regarding why it occurred. I then move to a consideration of several areas that may prove to be fruitful avenues of exploration for those who are grieving. The first such avenue is that of religion and spirituality as it relates to two concerns. I look at the way in which beliefs in this area may have proved inadequate, or may not even have been available, as well as the potential this domain offers for providing support. Next, I examine bibliotherapy, or the process of suggesting, selecting, and reading the stories of others who also have experienced the death of a loved one. The hope in this case is to provide a means by which the bereaved may both receive validation for present experiences and find guideposts for future searches. The third avenue of exploration to be addressed is that of death in other cultures. Accordingly, I consider the possibility that through an expansion of awareness about concepts subscribed to by others, those who mourn might find meaningful information for themselves. Finally, the chapter closes with a look at the process of writing new stories. This section includes some of the conclusions others have reached as well as a few of the ways in which we may aid those whom we desire to help to formulate their own ideas as they continue to engage in the process of searching for meaning.

THE DIMENSIONS OF THE DILEMMA

As discussed in Part I of the book, each type of death brings with it unique issues and concerns. Moreover, no two people respond to the same type of death in exactly the same way. Nevertheless, regardless of differences in reactions, always an underlying theme that emerges is the assault experienced by survivors on their view of reality. Always the world seems to look different after the death than it did before. Indeed, bereaved persons consistently report that, in one way or another, they found themselves rethinking much of what they formerly took for granted.

For example, when a parent loses a child, the death seems so unnatural, may be so bound up with feelings of guilt and failure (Rando, 1991), and may be so devastating to one's stability and everything in which one believed that it inevitably becomes the catalyst for a search for meaning. Whether the search is consciously or unconsciously undertaken, the parent undoubtedly will be assailed by conflicting emotions and numerous questions. What is more, the possibility of ever finding satisfactory answers may seem truly remote. As one mother describes her reactions, "I ranted and raved at a God I didn't believe in. How could He allow the most wonderful boy in the world, who was full of life yesterday, to be dead today?. . . How could He let this happen to me?. . . . My outraged soul screamed for answers to these questions even as I knew they would never come" (McCracken & Semel, 1998, p. 29).

Similarly, when a sibling dies, no matter at what age, there may be such a shattering of one's perspective that nothing seems to have meaning any longer. Though siblings may be reluctant, or may not have much opportunity, to speak of what is happening for them, there often is great turmoil seething beneath the appearance of equanimity as they simply go through the motions of living. A bereaved sister characterizes her experience as follows: "After my brother Bob's death, it seemed as though I had lost the capacity for emotional response. Daily life was in black and white, like a badly made film. My trancelike state excluded music, feeling, color, desire. Although on the surface I was doing well, I was actually going through each day like an automaton" (Conway, 1989, p. 121).

The death of one or both parents also is likely to shake the foundations on which the surviving children previously had built their lives. In this case, bereavement may include a great sense of aloneness and vulnerability along with grief. It also may bring a new comprehension of the role parents have played in protecting their children from some of life's harshest realities. The following quote illustrates feelings and insights such as these as expressed by a grieving daughter following the death of her father: "Dad's death challenged me to enter fully into the stream of life by shattering the world as I had known it and tearing down the boundaries I had carefully erected to feel more secure and in control. For weeks I longed for that illusion of security; I was amazed at how subtly my parents had buffered me from the deep realization of my own mortality, of the fragility of life, of my aloneness in the universe" (Kennedy, 1991, pp. 99–100).

In a like manner, when a spouse dies, the surviving husband or wife may feel totally lost and bewildered. He or she also is likely to experience, anger, frustration, and a loss of control. Though we may know, intellectually at least, that some day we, as spouses, eventually will be parted by death, emotionally we don't expect that day ever to come. According to one widow, "When your spouse dies, the lights go out. Your life may become dark, forlorn and dismal" (Zonnebelt-Smeenge & De Vries, 1998, p. 56).

Nor are we exempt from the attack on our view of reality when a close friend dies. Not only do we mourn the loss of a companion but we also may ponder such questions as why that person was chosen to die, who will be next, and how long each of us really has. Indeed, "The death of a friend can leave us staring into our own spiritual darkness" (Smith, 1996, p. 138). Thus, as with other kinds of losses, we confront similar kinds of fundamental doubts and concerns, those that are likely to shake up our world, impel us to delve deeply into our belief systems, and ultimately lead to vast changes in how we perceive reality. In other words, "Stressful events like bereavement require people to undertake a major revision of their assumptions and their ways of being in the world, and have long-lasting rather than transient implications" (Nolen-Hoeksema & Larson, 1999, p. 19).

In the immediate aftermath of the death, when it may be hard just to get through each day, the bereaved person is likely to alternate between doing nothing and questioning everything. In such a state, whatever answers are provided, or come too glibly from others, may not only be unsatisfactory but also may exacerbate feelings of hopelessness and helplessness. Indeed, just as the search for meaning tends to have long-lasting implications, it is a lengthy and painstaking process that evolves slowly. Further, the answers ideally must emerge from the experience of the bereaved person him- or herself, as he or she engages in such a process of exploration.

It is likely that in the beginning the primary focus will be on trying to figure out a cause for the death or on finding someone to blame (Shapiro, 1994). The immediate goal for most is to re-create a sense of the world as an orderly and predictable place, one in which they have some degree of control. Survivors therefore may blame themselves and/or second-guess their behavior prior to the death. For example, a widow whose husband died of a heart attack may wonder if she should have insisted that her spouse see a doctor. A friend may wonder what would have happened if he had not allowed a buddy to use his car and go out on the evening that the buddy died in a collision on an icy road. A mother may even ruminate about the events of the previous day and wonder if her daughter had had enough to eat the night before she died in freak accident. And many also turn outward in the attempt to find something or someone to blame.

In the case of death that is caused by illness, it thus is not unusual for bereaved persons to question the decisions of medical personnel or to become angry about treatments that did or did not take place. This is likely to happen even when everything done was medically appropriate. And in other cases, where there is a degree of culpability on the part of someone else, all the desolation and sadness felt by the bereaved person may be channeled into rage toward as well as a desire for vengeance relative to the guilty party. For example, a bereaved father spent many months plotting ways to harm the man who was driving the car that hit and killed his young daughter while she was crossing a street. However, in the long run, his feeling of impotence at not really being able to do anything to right the wrong only enhanced feelings of a world gone seriously awry.

When we lose a loved one, we ache for what was and what might have been. When we lose, as well, our meaning system, or a reason for being, it is little wonder that we feel utterly bereft. Indeed, "Although each person's meaning is different, existence that is merely a burden and lacks a future with any direction or point produces the worst kind of suffering" (Byock, 1997, p. 83). It is this kind of suffering to which we as helpers must become sensitive. And if we are to provide meaningful support, we also must be aware of various areas of belief that either may add to the burdens of the bereaved or offer the potential to provide solace. Thus, we turn now to a consideration of the varied roles played by religion and spirituality.

THE ROLE OF RELIGION AND SPIRITUALITY

For many people, religion and spirituality are a source of great comfort and support in their time of bereavement. Indeed, an increased observance of religious traditions may provide not only an important anchor but also a way to understand a divine purpose at work behind even the most tragic events (Schiff, 1977). Moreover, the set of rituals prescribed for dealing with death and mourning, as in the Jewish tradition, may help to bring a sense of order and predictability back into one's life.

However, one of the most typical responses of those who are bereaved is to become angry at a supposedly compassionate and benign God or Creator who could have allowed the death of a loved one (Bouvard & Gladu, 1998). This anger may emerge as a function of related beliefs that a life lived according to God's will or the precepts of a particular religious or spiritual tradition would serve as protection, thereby precluding the possibility of tragedy. For example, Rabbi Harold Kushner, in *When Bad Things Happen to Good People*, writes the following:

> Like most people, my wife and I had grown up with an image of God as an all-wise, all-powerful parent figure who would treat us as our earthly parents did, or even better. If we were obedient and deserving, He would reward us. If we got out of line, He would discipline us, reluctantly but firmly. He would protect us from being hurt or from hurting ourselves, and would see to it that we got what we deserved in life. (Kushner, 1981, p. 3)

However, when life happens, as it does, and the death of someone we love hurts us deeply, we cannot help but question such assumptions. Thus, depending on the extent of anger and disappointment at God, as well as the degree to which religion or spirituality formed an integral aspect of one's self-definition, a critical secondary loss may occur when a significant loss undermines one's faith (Rando, 1991). And even when ultimately our belief in God is not destroyed, we certainly may experience real disillusionment that a trusted belief system is not sufficient to provide the expected consolation. As a Christian theologian writes following the death of his son:

> Elements of the Gospel which I had always thought would console did not. They did something else, something important, but not that. It did not console me to be reminded of the hope of resurrection. If I had forgotten that hope, then it would indeed have brought light into my life to be reminded of it. But I did not think of death as a bottomless pit. I did not grieve as one who has no hope. Yet Eric is gone, *here* and *now* he is gone; *now* I cannot talk with him, *now* I cannot see him, *now* I cannot hug him, *now* I cannot hear of his plans for the future. *That* is my sorrow. A friend said, "Remember, he's in good hands." I was deeply moved. But that reality does not put Eric back in my hands now. That's my grief. For that grief, what consolation can there be other than having him back? (Wolterstorff, 1987, p. 31)

For those who consider themselves atheists or agnostics, different kinds of struggles may be initiated by the loss of a loved one. Such people have little to lean on or may experience the falling away of the last vestige of belief when a tragic death occurs. In the words of one mother following the death of her young son, "Jake's death nudged me off the fence of agnosticism on which I'd sat unconcerned for twenty years. It made me realize I was an atheist—confirmed but not angry. Some friends were incredulous that now, especially, I would reject the solace of religion" (McCracken & Semel, 1998, p. 30).

When we have no sense of a transcendent dimension, something larger than the self on whom or on which to rely, we are faced with the necessity for coming up with answers to the hard questions from within. In the instance of the mother just quoted, for example, the answer she ultimately accepted was that her son had been the victim of bad luck. Although such a conclusion may not be enough for some, for her it was the only one that seemed viable. However, whether the concepts and beliefs of a religious or spiritual tradition are either being seriously questioned or simply are not relevant sources of support, there is much that others can do to assist the search for meaning in this area.

Indeed, the greatest help may be provided just by listening carefully and offering questions and reflections that test the logic of various lines of reasoning. Although we may not share similar beliefs, perhaps our request for explanations may enable those we desire to help to become clearer in their thinking. When our belief systems are related or we have had comparable experiences, we may offer what we have learned and what we now believe as food for thought. And we can share knowledge about the beliefs subscribed to by members of different religious and spiritual traditions. Thus we may act as midwives for the birthing of new or revised meaning systems.

We also may make contact with or refer those who are bereaved to members of the clergy or other spiritual leaders when greater expertise seems appropriate. We may recommend a retreat or workshop focusing on the religious or spiritual dimension. We thus may give permission for a wider search. In addition, we may recommend books that help those who are bereaved as they struggle with questions related to this area. What is more, although books may be an important resource in the quest for understanding relative to religion and spirituality, the use of bibliotherapy also may prove useful in many other areas related to the search for meaning.

BIBLIOTHERAPY

Suggesting particular books, and perhaps also videotapes, to supplement therapy sessions is common practice in the mental health field. Resources such as these provide information in a different format and may be accessed at a pace that is chosen by each person. However, bibliotherapy may be especially helpful when working with those who are grieving. As noted in Chapter 6, parents who have lost a child may be especially interested in and helped by reading about the experiences of other parents whose child has died. For example, a bereaved father writes, "I do appreciate learning about the struggle of others, the questions they have faced, and how their cry has been met" (Strommen & Strommen, 1993, p. 19). In addition to helping bereaved parents, reading may be an important avenue of exploration for those who are bereaved as a function of many other kinds of loss.

It therefore may be appropriate to be familiar with various resources available and to be able to recommend specific books or tapes for different kinds of situations. For example, one of my favorites for dealing with grief in the weeks immediately following a death, and for gathering enough strength to want to continue living, is titled *To Heal Again* (Berkus, 1984). This is a beautifully illustrated book with many pictures and few words. Each page may be contemplated as a separate meditation or the entire book may be read easily in one sitting. The message to be kind to oneself, to take the necessary time to recover and to trust that healing will come seems extremely important to me. It also is a book that might be suitable for many in that though there is a spiritual undertone, the author does not seem to make recourse to any one religious tradition.

For others, books with a particular religious focus, one in which the author wrestles with the precepts of a particular tradition, may be useful as the bereaved person begins the process of confronting his or her spiritual doubts and questions. In this regard, *A Grief Observed* by C. S. Lewis (1976) is probably the classic for those whose orientation is Christian. The movie *Shadowlands*, which is based on Lewis's book, might also prove helpful either as a supplement to the book or as a substitute for those who prefer to watch rather than read. In *The Bereaved Parent*, Harriet Sarnoff Schiff (1977) includes in her chapter on bereavement and religion some of her experiences and thoughts as a member of the Jewish tradition. Throughout the rest of the book she also offers some wise and helpful insights on a variety of additional topics.

As mentioned previously, many who are bereaved also want some confirmation that life continues after death, that their loved ones survive in some way, that future contact may be possible. From traditional philosophical and religious discussions to an exploration of out-of-body, near-death, and psychic experiences, the list of possible books related to this topic is endless. Indeed, as a person moves into this realm, it may be better to suggest a strategy for discovery rather than the titles of particular books. Accordingly, I recommend that the bereaved person go to a library or bookstore and just browse, waiting to get an intuitive sense about what would be most appropriate to read. From there, I suggest a snowball process, where one book or idea leads to another. As I offer this strategy, I often use my own experience as an illustration.

After my son's death, the first books I read were those given to me by friends and they focused mainly on the stories of other parents who had lost children. I found them as helpful as anything else offered to me at that time. Eventually, however, it became necessary for me to find some books on my own. Because I was in a university context, and because I like to own my books, I decided to go to the campus bookstore to locate additional reading material. While there, I wandered around and picked out several possible books but then decided to reject most of them. However, there was one that for some reason or other I simply couldn't put back on the shelf. Each time I tried, I would have second thoughts. So I bought it.

Although the book *Talking with Nature* (Roads, 1985) was not about death or grief, it opened many doors to a realm still very new to me at that time—that of metaphysics. Indeed, it turned out to be a wonderful choice. After reading this book it seemed as though there were no holds barred and each one I read quickly led to another. The books I initially chose included some with such unlikely titles as *Death Brings Many Surprises* (Coddington, 1987), *Life between Death and Rebirth* (Steiner, 1968), *Life between Life* (Whitton & Fisher, 1986), *The Dead Are Alive* (Sherman, 1981), and *The New Thought Christian* (Warch, 1977). I also began reading the personal reports of others who had explored the metaphysical realm. Over the years, my journey has included hundreds of books on a vast array of topics. Indeed, reading for me is a source of enormous comfort as well as information in my continuing efforts to understand life and to live comfortably with death.

However, any process of discovery through reading will undoubtedly lead in as many different directions, with as many different variations, as there are people searching. Given the overwhelming number of books available, and their even easier access today because of the Internet, what is important is to help bereaved persons find or create a strategy that facilitates their quest for meaning. And in addition to a useful strategy as well as information relative to the topics already mentioned, we as professionals also may offer further suggestions regarding other areas on which to focus. One that may be extremely helpful following the loss of a loved one pertains to attempts undertaken from the perspective of various cultures to understand death. And although explorations in this area may include books and tapes, they certainly may move into other modalities as well.

EXPLORING DEATH IN OTHER CULTURES

One aspect of the dilemma of death for those of us who live in Western society is the acceptance of a linear rather than a circular worldview. Consistent with such a view, we tend to believe that we are born and then we die. And although most philosophical and religious traditions, both Western and Eastern, have included from earliest history a concept of the soul as an animating principal (Raheem, 1991), and the "immortality of the soul is the most essential concept of all religions" (Achte, 1980), in our society we certainly do not generally subscribe to the idea of repeating lifetimes in a physical incarnation. Indeed, we are not even much inclined to integrate the realms of life and death:

> In this century, at least for Americans, connection between the world of the dead and that of the living has been largely severed and the dead world is disappearing. Communion between the two realms has come to an end. It is a radical departure because for three centuries prior, life and death were not held apart. Meaning flowed freely between the two worlds. It is radical also in that the movement toward withdrawal from the dead reversed a strong trend apparent through most of the nineteenth century, in which the place and role of the dead in the world of the living was increasing significantly. (Jackson, 1980, p. 47)

Not only have we in U.S. society changed our general attitudes about death, but as we consider the belief systems of both other cultures and earlier manifestations within our own culture we find that reincarnation also was a concept that was once widely accepted (Sogyal, 1992). What is more, it continues to be an important belief in many societies today. What may be reassuring in all this for those who have experienced the death of a loved one is the discovery that there are many ways to understand what happens after we die. Also a source of consolation may be the idea that the survivor and the one who has died will be together again, either physically or in the afterlife. And there may be something very exciting, and perhaps confirming, about finding extremely similar descriptions of what happens after we die from the perspective of two or more very different cultures or worldviews.

The idea of reincarnation certainly is not for everyone, and indeed might be threatening for many, but after a death people often show a greater willingness to search beyond previously established limits. When old concepts do not provide enough support, the search for new ones becomes appropriate. Thus, bereaved persons may be encouraged not only to read about the traditions of other cultures but also to go exploring in a variety of ways. In addition to finding books, attending a workshop or enrolling in a course may prove helpful. Becoming involved with a group consisting of like-minded individuals desiring to learn about another tradition also may aid the search process. For example, in our current era there is much interest in, and therefore many opportunities for exploration of, both Eastern and Native American belief systems. Regardless of the path taken, however, ultimately what may be most important is assistance with the process of integrating new information into old frames of reference and thereby writing new stories which enable us to once again experience life in a meaningful way.

WRITING NEW STORIES

It is a truism, however trite, that every ending is also a beginning. No matter how much against our will, the death of someone we love ends a chapter even as it also initiates another. However, although the pain may seem unbearable and the devastation too great, the potential for healing and transformation greater than we could possibly imagine not only exists but is an outcome that is universally typical: "Wounding often involves a painful excursion into pathos; we experience massive anguish, and the suffering cracks the boundaries of what we thought we could stand. And yet, time and again, I discover that the wounding pathos of our own local stories contain the seeds of healing and even of transformation. This truth is woven into all classic tales of the human condition" (Houston, 1996, p. 267).

The local stories that each of us participates in writing for ourselves become the reality we inhabit, living us as much as we live it:

> Stories are habitations. We live in and through stories. They conjure worlds. We do not know the world other than as story world. Stories inform life. They hold us together and keep us apart. We inhabit the great stories of our culture. We live through stories. We are lived by the stories of our race and place. It is this enveloping and constituting function of stories that is especially important to sense more fully. We are, each of us, locations where the stories of our place and time become partially tellable. (Mair, 1988, p. 127)

Given their importance in creating and sustaining reality, if the stories that provided the foundation on which we lived are destroyed or become outmoded, it is essential that we adapt our tales to fit the conditions that now define our experience as human beings. Indeed, even as we accept the challenges entailed with exploration, with the search for greater understanding, we have begun the process of rewriting our life stories. Ultimately, however, the time may come when it is important to focus on the integration of all that has been learned while acknowledging that new chapters will inevitably require further revisions.

For some, the new story may not require or involve the overhaul of an entire belief system. Rather, some sense of peace may be achieved through a simple reevaluation process. For example, "More than one grieving parent has found meaning in balancing the sense of tragedy by considering the time they had together as a precious gift" (Byock, 1997, p. 281). Others, by contrast, may find meaning only through investing themselves in a cause, although even the nature of the cause may change over the years. As the founder of MADD writes 10 years after beginning this organization:

> I have realized that for me, finding fulfillment means being committed to an issue. Although I will always care about the issue of drunk driving, I've become very concerned about the issue of victims of violent crime during the last three years. . . . I also have other interests. I'm concerned about the stereotyping of Arab-Americans, about discrimination against them, and about peace in the Middle East. (Lightner & Hathaway, 1990, p. 229)

Similarly, as bereaved persons focus on the new stories that are being written it is not at all unusual for them to choose to make career changes; to participate in different kinds of activities, hobbies, or interests; to feel more concerned about expressing themselves more creatively (Brooks, 1999). And for some, the extent of change in perceptions may be so great that they are reluctant to share their new views with others. They may be surprised themselves at what they have come to believe and certainly recognize the skepticism of others given the radical shift their worldview has undergone (Rothschild, 2000). As one who has had such an experience writes: "This is, quite frankly, a lot to believe: friendships and conversations, begun here, resumed in eternity with little notice of a pause? Surely you don't really believe that? Well, it's one of those ideas that I have chosen not to be too vocal about. I want neither to be challenged nor dismissed. I simply need this belief" (Smith, 1996, p. 128).

Indeed, what is important is that the belief works. Whether it is true or false is not nearly as crucial as whether it helps us make sense of loss, adjust to pain, and move to a place where happiness and sorrow are able to coexist—for the ultimate goal of helping families to successfully resolve death, dying, bereavement, and related end-of-life issues, as well as facilitating their processes of searching for meaning, is attainment of the ability to reclaim joy as a valid part of life.

THERAPEUTIC CONVERSATIONS
AND REFLECTIONS

∾

A young man in his early 40s had come to therapy seeking help with career decisions. He was married, had two young children, and in the eyes of the world would certainly have been considered successful. However, although he had pursued several different avenues in the work world and certainly had done well financially over the years, a feeling of satisfaction always had eluded him. Others thought he was crazy to continue the pattern of doubting what he was doing and his wife worried about the family and their security each time he made a job change. His own fear was that he would continue this pattern without finding what he was searching for and that as an old man he would regret the choices he had made or had not made.

In the effort to help him achieve his goal of finding a career he would experience as satisfying, one that enabled him to have a sense of purpose beyond financial gain, we explored several areas. We considered the family in which he grew up and the paths that others whom he respected had chosen for themselves. We considered as well the messages he had received from parents and teachers regarding his talents and what significant others felt it would be most appropriate for him to pursue. We discussed the interests and activities in which he had invested time and energy both as a child and later in life. We compared his lifestyle and work choices with those of classmates and friends. And we focused a great deal of energy on sorting out what a sense of purpose meant for him, when he had experienced it in the past, in however small a way, and what might be going on for him if it occurred again in the future.

During the course of our conversations, my client described an incident that he believed had had a tremendous impact on him and yet one whose full import he had never before seriously examined. That is, while in college he had had a close friend with whom he spent a great deal of time. They participated on sports teams together, they went camping together, and they both delighted in orchestrating practical jokes which they perpetrated on friends. More important, however, this friend had been not only a truly good person but also someone who was deeply spiritual. He had had a real sense of mission about what he intended to accomplish in his life. His goal was to help children and to that end he planned to go to medical school and then to move to a Third World country where he felt his services would be most needed and thus of the greatest value. Shortly after graduation from college, however, the friend had been diagnosed with cancer and within 6 months had died.

My client knew nothing of the illness or his friend's death until several months after it had occurred. The reason for this was that following graduation he had decided to travel in Europe and it wasn't until he returned home that he learned what had happened. He was stunned to hear the news and angry at himself for having been out of touch for so long. What is more, those who had gathered for the funeral had dispersed and he had few with whom he could talk about what had happened. He therefore felt there was nothing to do except go on with his life. Although he continued to think about and to miss his friend, he mainly became caught up in concerns related to jobs, marriage, children, and family.

As he recounted this story, my client began to cry. He cried for his friend, for the injustice that the life of such a good person had been cut so short, for his own lack of understanding about how this could have happened. He also cried for himself as he began to recognize that what he longed for was the feeling that had been so important to his friend—that he had a mission to accomplish in this life.

Although he certainly was not interested in becoming a physician, my client also began to recognize a desire to in some way participate in achieving his friend's goal of helping children. As we explored various ways in which to do that, it became clear that a career change would not necessarily be required. Rather, there were many charitable activities in which he could become involved. Indeed, his financial resources enabled him to provide a great deal of help through contributions of both time and money. Although this seemed to be sufficient initially, eventually my client decided to return to graduate school and today works as a social worker in a treatment center for abused children.

It is interesting for me to consider the effect the friend's death had on the life of my client, even years after the loss occurred. It is also critical to consider how, although not conscious, there was an awareness of something unsettled that continued to brew under the surface for many years. Indeed, it was this very sense that something was missing, and more important that somehow it was related to his friend, that ultimately demanded attention as it emerged into consciousness. And it is intriguing to recognize how an event so seemingly meaningless as the death of a fine young man also became the catalyst that, in this instance, provided crucial information that enabled resolution in the search for meaning.

CHAPTER 13

Reclaiming Joy

My husband and I met in college and married soon after we both graduated. We shared many similar interests, including a love of the outdoors and camping as well as a desire to have a large family. We were a good fit, content just spending time together and also comfortable when one or the other needed time alone. We were anxious to become parents and much to our delight, our first child was born a year and a half after we were married. Our second child, another daughter, arrived on schedule 2 years later. My husband was doing well in his work and I was happy to be able to be a stay-at-home mom. We had hoped to have at least two more children, but just prior to our fifth wedding anniversary, my husband was diagnosed with cancer.

To say that we were terribly frightened by this dreadful disease does not begin to convey the magnitude of our panic and shock. Somehow the hand of fate, or of God, had dealt us an unbelievable blow and we were anything but prepared. We had been so happy with our two beautiful little girls and the life we had been intent on creating. Suddenly, however, all our plans seemed to have been for naught and everything about life appeared to be up for grabs.

In the first 2 years after the diagnosis it took most of our energy just to get through the treatments and deal with numerous hospitalizations while trying to maintain some semblance of normality for our children. At the same time, we were determined that we were going to get through this nightmare and win the battle for my husband's life. And for a long time, we did. Eventually my husband went into remission and what followed were 4 years of a fairly normal life. Of course, the black cloud of cancer seemed always to hang over our heads and each checkup was faced with fear, which continued until the results of various tests confirmed that things were still going well.

The children knew that their daddy had been very sick and they were sensitive to changes in our moods that could be triggered even when he just had a cold. But for the most part we did a good job of creating a stable and happy home life. My husband went back to work and I was able to participate in activities at my daughters' schools. Once again, the children seemed to be thriving and we had so much for which to be grateful. Indeed, we felt truly blessed and we tried to live each minute of each day to the fullest. As it turned out, these posttreatment years were some of the happiest of my life and I suspect that they were for my husband as well.

Unfortunately for all of us, however, the day did come when the cancer returned. And once again we fought it with every bit of energy we could muster. Despite severely debilitating and sometimes experimental treatments, my husband hung in there and continued to be optimistic. And this struggle bought us 4 more years. However, these years were like a constant roller-coaster ride with our emotions going from high to low and back again as he attempted to fight his way back to health and reassure himself and us that everything would turn out OK. But in the end, he just wasn't able to beat the odds, his body gave out and the cancer won.

When my husband died, we had been living with cancer, on and off, for 10 years. At some level, I always knew there was a possibility that he would die. But I had never allowed myself to believe it would really happen. Oh, we had prepared our wills and done all the appropriate legal things, but I just felt like that was a precaution. It was almost like a preventive measure, like carrying an umbrella so it won't rain. My husband's optimism also had convinced me—and I had wanted to be convinced—that we would enjoy old age together. But we were wrong.

When he died, I thought my life was over as well. Oh yes, I still had my children but a world without my beloved husband was almost more than I could comprehend. I did what needed to be done in terms of arranging for the funeral, dealing with the kids, answering the phone, whatever. But it was as though I was in a fog and I couldn't see or think clearly about anything.

Some weeks later, I remember a friend taking me out with her for the day and I just followed along, blindly, not sure where we were or what we were doing. The nights were even worse and sleep offered little comfort. I would go to bed and feel so terribly cold but no matter how many quilts and blankets I piled on, I just couldn't seem to get warm.

I also hurt physically. It felt like I had been kicked in the chest and I realized what it really meant to have a broken heart. My husband and I had been so close and now he was so far away. Our connection, the wonderful bond of love that we had shared, seemed to have been severed and the pain was as real as if my body actually had been wounded. I couldn't eat, I couldn't sleep and if it hadn't been for the children I'm not sure what I would have done. I previously had never been able to fathom how a person could even contemplate, let alone *actually commit, suicide. Now I understood, although in truth this was never really a viable option for me.*

After several months I began meeting with the pastor of our church, who was also trained as a therapist, and he encouraged me to start attending services. Although my husband and I had made sporadic attempts over the years to take our children to Sunday school, we had not really been church-goers ourselves. We had had the children baptized and we had gone during the holidays like Christmas and Easter, but we just had not been particularly interested in becoming more involved. I now began to go more regularly even though, at first, being in church just made me cry. There was something about the music—perhaps it was the association with my husband's funeral—that seemed to unleash my tears. Nevertheless, like so many things I did during that period in my life, I at least went through the motions even when my heart certainly was far from being in the activity.

In time, I met some wonderful people through the church and several of them now have become close friends. I am grateful for their presence in my life because so many of the friends my husband and I had while he was alive are no longer part of my world. Yes, some of our couple friends tried to include me in social gatherings in the beginning, but often I refused. Or, if I would go, I just felt so awkward and uncomfortable that it just was not worth the effort. But many others just seemed to forget about me, which still makes me very angry when I think about it.

However, I did slowly begin to participate more at my church, particularly with various programs for children. After several years I became a Sunday school teacher and even helped to rewrite the curriculum for the entire church school. In fact, I became so interested in education that when my daughters were both in high school, I decided to go back and get a master's degree and to become certified as an elementary school teacher. Today I work at the school my daughters attended when they were younger.

It has been 7 years since my husband died and so much has changed. In addition to finding a career, I also decided to sell our old house and move to a newer, smaller one that was more manageable for me and a little closer to where I work. My older daughter has graduated from college and is now in law school. She is engaged to a wonderful young man and plans to be married once she has completed her education and has found a job. My younger daughter is in college, majoring in psychology and enjoying a variety of extracurricular activities. Although very different, each has become a beautiful young woman and they are very protective of each other. I know how proud my husband would be if he were here to see them.

I still cry easily and often, especially at occasions like graduations or activities in which my daughters are participants because it seems so unfair that their father is not here to share these events with us. His birthday and the anniversary of his death are also particularly challenging, although each year it seems to get a little easier. Until now I have been very focused on supporting my children and finding something that makes life seem more meaningful to me. And for a long time, I simply thought that I probably would never marry again. I was so happy, so blessed, in my first marriage that I have doubted that I could ever find another person with whom I would want to share my life. However, that is beginning to change.

Although my life is good, and I am content, I am aware that I would prefer not to be alone forever. My daughters will soon be out on their own and I am still relatively young. So, my thoughts have turned to the possibility of dating. At first I felt really guilty about the idea of being with someone else. It seemed as though I was betraying my husband and what we had together. But when I think about it realistically, I am sure that he would want me to be happy. At the same time, in some ways it is easier to stay safely inside the little world I have created for myself. Although I have begun to attend dances with single friends, I feel terribly awkward when approached by another man. It almost feels like I am back in high school again, and I don't enjoy the feelings now any more than I did then. Fortunately, I'm not in any hurry to find another husband and am willing to wait and see what happens.

In the meantime, I feel very proud of what I have been able to accomplish. I think I will always miss my husband, will always feel that somehow we were cheated. I probably will never understand why things turned out as they did. But I can honestly say that I am happy with my life, at least for the most part. I now know that the bond that my husband and I shared in life continues even in death, because I sometimes feel his presence. I also am aware that I have done things I probably would never have attempted if he had lived and I feel like he is cheering me on. At the same time, I know that I am more realistic than I once was. I allow myself to cry when I feel like it but I also am no longer afraid to enjoy myself or think about the future in a positive way, despite my reluctance to do this in the beginning. Surprisingly enough, I am once again excited about the adventure of life and look forward to many more years. Hopefully they will bring with them more understanding, acceptance and greater joy for all of us.

—AN

Just as life and death represent logical complementarities as discussed in Chapter 1, or are two sides of the same conceptual coin, so also are joy and sorrow. That is, we cannot make sense of or truly understand one notion, or one side of the coin, without the other as a contrast with which to

compare it. And despite the fact that we might choose to have it be otherwise, all—life/death, joy/sorrow—are integral parts of our experience as
human beings. Or in the witty but nevertheless wise words of the poet
William Blake (cited in *Oxford Dictionary of Quotations*, 1980, p. 85):

> A truth that's told with bad intent
> Beats all the lies you can invent.
> It is right it should be so;
> Man was made for Joy and Woe;
> And when this we rightly know,
> Thro' the World we safely go,
> Joy and woe are woven fine,
> A clothing for the soul divine.

What is more, not only are "joy and woe" conceptually inseparable as well
as finely woven together in the fabric of life, thus providing "clothing for
the soul divine," but the experience of each also enhances the knowledge
of the other, thereby enriching our ability to live more fully.

However, in our society we seem to expect only joy, we expect things
always to go well. We never ask "Why me?" when pleasurable things happen. We don't investigate the causes of our good fortune. When we encounter happiness, it feels like our birthright and we therefore take it and
run. On the other hand, when disappointment and loss occur we immediately start to question a cruel fate that has brought sadness into our world.
We don't understand that this, too, is an inevitable and equally valuable
part of life. And because of such a stance, we not only feel sad but we label
such experiences as bad. By so doing, however, we fail to honor and respect grief both as the lifelong companion it is likely to become and as the
bearer not only of great sorrow and woe but also, at least potentially, of
many gifts, including the ability truly to know joy.

There is no question in my mind that losing someone you dearly love
and to whom you were deeply attached is one of the most painful and hor-
rifying events any of us will ever have to endure. Similarly, I know that
the healing journey is long and tortuous, with many stops and starts and a
multitude of turns in the road. I recognize that, at least at the outset, the
idea of ever being happy again may be so remote as to seem ridiculous. Indeed, there may be seemingly insurmountable obstacles to overcome as
part of the quest for the resolution of grief and all its attendant issues.
Along the way we may grow weary and, to add to our pain, others may decide they no longer wish to accompany us. Nevertheless, I believe it is im-

portant to remember that none of this defines the journey as inherently bad. What is more, I am convinced that no other experience has the capacity for teaching us more about ourselves and others than does creating life and striving to reclaim joy in the presence of grief.

To reclaim joy, however, does not mean that a constant state of euphoria is ever achieved or even to be desired. Rather, it means that the bereaved person takes whatever measures are necessary to grieve fully and to allow healing to occur—however long it takes and whatever is required to do so. It means facing and dealing with the secondary losses that may accompany a death as well as with the feelings that are likely to be evoked by such losses. It means overcoming the barriers that threaten one's sense of well-being as they continue to elicit sadness and tears long after the death. It means allowing new parts of the self to emerge in order to accommodate the new world that one has entered and is in an ongoing process of recreating. It means permitting oneself to be happy again, perhaps learning to live at two levels (Becvar, 1997), and recognizing that one can simultaneously acknowledge both joy and sorrow. It means being able, finally, to understand what it really means to be "joy-full."

The discussions in this concluding chapter therefore focus on three major areas. The first of these deals with overcoming specific obstacles, or barriers to healing, faced by those who are bereaved. Additional suggestions that may guide professionals in their efforts to help family members effectively resolve such issues as anger, guilt, unresolved conflicts, and the repair and reconstruction of belief systems thus are provided. Vulnerability to illness and the importance of self-care on the part of those who are grieving are considered. Also included are some ways in which to foster a sense of connection between bereaved persons and their loved ones who have died as well as suggestions for preparations in this area before the death has occurred. In the second section I define and discuss what it means to live at two levels and how it is possible to take a both/and perspective that enables one to embrace and live simultaneously with both happiness and sadness. In addition, I examine some of the challenges entailed with rebuilding a life as well as with attempts to find or understand the logic of what has happened. Other issues to be considered are those related to accepting the many losses that accompany the death of a loved one, including interactions with others in one's world. In the third and final section I consider the gifts of grief and the ways in which, despite the pain, life may be enriched as a function of the loss. Such potential gifts include an enhanced ability to be compassionate and tolerant, greater awareness and valuing of life, loss of the fear of death, and appreciation, once again, of the sights and sounds of our world. Indeed, by way of conclusion, I consider the possibility that a whole new sense of peace and serenity relative to life and living may be acquired in the process of reclaiming joy.

OVERCOMING BARRIERS TO HEALING

I have noted throughout, and particularly as it relates to parents who have lost a child, the importance for family members of the opportunity to tell their story. Thus, for example, we may recognize that sharing stories of their loss may provide emotional relief for bereaved persons at the same time that it encourages the search for meaning (Sedney, Baker, & Gross, 1994). In addition, it may help to bring family members closer together as they hear and are able to understand each other more clearly. And others who are privileged to be able to listen to these stories also may gather information about the way each person constructs her or his narrative, or view of reality.

Indeed, as part of the recounting of events, problematic areas, those in which assistance might be appropriate and meaningful, also may be highlighted. For example, various unresolved issues such as guilt, blame, or a feeling of responsibility relative to the death may emerge as significant impediments to the recovery process. Having identified such stumbling blocks, helpers may be able to focus particularly in these areas.

Not only does the opportunity to share stories have the potential to provide new and potentially useful information, but it also may encourage feelings of competency and control for the narrators. What is more, it may enable everyone involved to offer support, to help alleviate whatever anxiety individuals may be experiencing, and thereby enhance a feeling of connectedness. Finally, change may be monitored and noted as new ideas are incorporated into old stories, shifts in emphasis evolve and different meanings are created. Ideally, when the sharing of stories is used as part of therapy with bereaved families, "the death comes to be viewed as an experience that the family can talk about, cope with, and incorporate into their ongoing family story. The focus is on respect for each individual's unique experience within a family context" (Sedney et al., 1994, p. 294).

The process of sharing stories also may be expanded on by inviting bereaved persons to write down their narratives and then perhaps read what they have written aloud. Although not appropriate for everyone, writing for some may be a means of bringing order to scattered thoughts and feelings. In addition, such an approach may enable others to get a more concrete sense of core beliefs, some of which also may be barriers to healing. Indeed, whether in written or oral form, understanding how various persons construe their reality (Kelly, 1955) is essential to the ability of others to provide information that may be meaningful, information that may open doors to new beliefs and behaviors and thus may facilitate change.

A further useful variation on the theme of storytelling may be that of having some or all the participants write and then read to one another their reflections on the experience of therapy. Whether the goal is an informal sharing of information or a formal manuscript to be submitted for publication (e.g., Levac, McLean, Wright, & Bell, 1998), healing may be the outcome. Thus, what may be most helpful is the opportunity such an approach provides to clarify perceptions and correct perceived misunderstandings on the part of both professionals and other family members.

Another barrier to healing may arise as a function of the fact that the most recent death is yet one more in a series of losses. For example, a young woman recently referred to me for therapy has suffered in the last 5 years the accidental death of her brother, the murder of her mother, and the death of a friend to cancer. Though in this instance the degree of loss is immediately apparent, often it is not. Therefore, it may become important to map patterns over several generations of a family in order to "locate epicenters of trauma and loss" (Horwitz, 1997, p. 215). One then may focus on understanding previous attempts by family members to resolve their grief as well as any remaining issues related to past losses. This information then may be used to help alleviate the pain that currently is being experienced.

Another particularly challenging hurdle may be present in the cases of those whose loved ones died in such a manner that they were severely disfigured or were the victims of some form of trauma or brutality. Deeply distressing images and/or frightening thoughts about how the deceased persons looked or what they may have experienced before dying are likely to haunt the bereaved, adding significantly to the stress of the loss. In this case, the use of guided imagery may be appropriate as a possible aid to healing. Following some instructions to gently relax the entire body, the bereaved client is invited first to see the deceased person at the time of death and then, gradually, through a focus on sending love and healing energy, to transform the image. The ultimate goal is for the client to be able to hold in her or his mind's eye a view of the loved one as healthy and normal, thus transforming the negative image into one that is positive. Further, by offering an opportunity to participate in "healing" the one who has died, such a process also may enable the client to move beyond the distressing thoughts and concerns that previously were a major preoccupation and/or focus of rumination.

Also recommended for situations of traumatic loss and unresolved grief is the approach known as eye movement desensitization and reprocessing (EMDR; Solomon & Shapiro, 1997). Following a carefully structured treatment protocol, EMDR involves (1) taking a history, (2) preparing the client, (3) assessing the target of the intervention, (4) desensitizing negative affect, (5) enhancing positive cognitions, (6) scanning the body for residual tension, (7) closing the session, and (8) reevaluation. However, although potentially useful, EMDR requires specialized training. Therefore, knowledge of appropriately prepared professionals to whom one may make referrals is essential should such an approach be deemed desirable and appropriate.

On the other hand, thought field therapy (Callahan & Callahan, 1997) requires no specialized training for those who desire to use it in their efforts to help bereaved persons deal with their grief. This process involves teaching clients to tap on specific body points while focusing on upsetting emotions and at the same time engaging in activities such as moving their eyes, humming, or counting. It is a procedure that is individualized for each client and "the emphasis of therapy is on the effort to help the bereaved become as strong as possible in the face of the tragedy and to facilitate the wholesome survival of the family" (Callahan & Callahan, 1997, p. 255).

Regardless of the circumstances of the death, somatic complaints and sometimes serious illness also may occur in the aftermath of a significant loss. It therefore behooves helpers to assess sleep patterns, dietary habits, and the degree of support available as well as ways in which the bereaved person is or is not taking care of him- or herself. Gentle exercise, particularly walking, may be helpful antidotes to both disturbances with sleep and depressed moods. Depending on the severity in either area, a referral to a physician also may be in order. Similarly, loss of appetite and lack of interest in food, though normal in the beginning, may warrant further attention should the pattern continue for a prolonged period of time. What is more, being aware of the need to eat healthy food may be extremely important during the early phases of bereavement and the support of others, when available, may be enlisted in this regard. Finally, appropriate self-care also means allowing regular time for tears, learning to go day by day, and understanding that the process usually involves taking two steps forward and one step backward—that relapses are normal and certainly will occur.

A final obstacle to be overcome may be that of achieving some sense of connection with the deceased person. Indeed, the idea that a relationship has simply ended may be so unacceptable as to be debilitating for some. Therefore, it may be important to support or help bereaved persons in this area, understanding that far from being a stumbling block to the resolution of grief, a sense that the relationship continues may be extremely healing (Klass, Silverman, & Nickman, 1996). Various ways to help in this regard have been discussed throughout the book, ranging from awareness of fond memories to a sense of an interactive relationship. However, we return to the topic once again in acknowledgment of the potential for healing that may be derived from understanding "that survivors hold the deceased in loving memory for long periods, often forever, and that maintaining an inner representation of the deceased is normal rather than abnormal" (Silverman & Nickman, 1996, p. 349). In some instances, the establishment of such a connection may be prepared for and enhanced before a person dies.

That is, in the case of an anticipated death, the making of videotapes (Rigazio-DiGilio, 2001), whether of therapy sessions, of shared interactions at home or in order to create personal messages to be shared with others, may provide wonderful opportunities both to facilitate the dying process and to create a visual legacy for the future. In the course of their creation, those with a terminal illness have an opportunity to derive new meanings from the re-creation of their life stories. Some of the specific needs of clients which may be met through such a process include finishing previously unfinished business, allowing the dying person to live more fully, creating an atmosphere in which everyone may say good-bye, fostering a context for bereavement, and prompting reexamination of developmental issues and tasks. What is more, when completed, "these videos allow the client's story to live on, even for family members not yet born, thus reinforcing the continuity of family history. For friends, cherished memories and images of the departed, or of a particular collection of individuals will be preserved throughout their lifetime. And for the community, new persuasive ideas might be encapsulated in these videos" (Rigazio-DiGilio, 2001).

For those dealing with sudden death, other means of achieving similar ends may include making a video which includes survivors telling their stories about the person and is interspersed with pictures of the deceased and/or with clips of videos made prior to the death. Regardless of the method, finding ways to maintain a sense of a continuing presence, as well as acknowledgment that the one who died really did live and have an impact on others, may be very healing. It also may be important to the achievement of feelings of connection to the deceased person as well as to the creation of a story that supports such feelings. What is more, attaining this sense of a continuing bond or relationship may be one extremely important aspect of the process of living at two levels.

LIVING AT TWO LEVELS

As described elsewhere (Becvar, 1997), living at two levels means being able to acknowledge and access simultaneously both the domain of the material, or the biological, and the domain of the intangible, or the spiritual. We may think of the former as our normal, everyday physical reality, the one we come to know and understand as a function of information gathered through the senses of sight, smell, hearing, touch, and taste. The latter refers to a paranormal, nontangible, reality, knowledge of which we must gather intuitively, or through faith, as we acknowledge and make recourse to a belief in a larger, transcendent dimension:

> There are indeed fundamentally two categories of knowledge—Knowledge by Ideation and Knowledge by Being. All scientific knowledge, whether physical or super-physical, belongs to the first category. Such knowledge is based on the duality of the observer and observed. In spiritual perception, however, there is Knowledge by Being—it arises in that state where the duality of the observer and the observed has vanished. This is the very core of direct or what is otherwise called the Mystical Experience. (Mehta, 1967, p. 7)

However, though "Knowledge by Being" may be the core of mystical experience, one does not have to be a mystic in order to experience it. Nor does one have to be religious. Rather, as one has a sense of the presence of a person who has died, of a soul whose existence continues beyond death, one has accessed the level of the spiritual. This may occur through direct contact, through trust in synchronistic events, or simply through faith in an enduring and ongoing relationship which may never be confirmed in any tangible way.

Each person who grieves, of course, must learn how to continue to live in and survive successfully in the material or biological realm. At the same time, a major preoccupation is likely to be with thoughts about what has happened to the person following death. Through awareness of the spiritual, or nonphysical, level of being, the bereaved person may achieve some measure of acceptance. And such acceptance may lead to a sense of peace and serenity even as the person faces the terrible pain associated with the loss of the physical presence of the one who has died.

As one is able to balance and hold in awareness these two levels of reality one also may be more successful in attempts to come to terms with, or to understand the logic of, what has occurred. For example, in the immediate aftermath of my son's death, I could make or find absolutely no sense in what to me was an utter tragedy. To my logical mind, there was simply no reason why a fine young man in the prime of life, a good person with vast potential, should suddenly and violently have lost his life. Nor could I understand what we, his family, had done to deserve the suffering that his loss created. In time, however, as I achieved greater awareness and acceptance of what I call the spiritual dimensions of life in general, and of my son's death in particular, I was able to create a story that felt "true" for me and thus brought me a great deal of peace.

Specifically, I began to believe more fully in the degree to which we participate in creating our reality, including the choice of when and how we die. That is, I accepted the idea that we all have a mission, or a purpose created a soul level, to fulfill while we live and that learning and growth are the ultimate goals for each of us. When we complete in each lifetime whatever small part of this goal it was we came to do, we move on, or die. Thus, I also began to embrace the idea that in order to achieve the totality of our goals, we live many lives—the idea of reincarnation. What is more, I came to believe that as we live again and again we often do so with the same people. That is, we travel in soul groups. With this story I was able to accept that in a larger, more encompassing reality my son's death was somehow "appropriate" even though in the reality in which I live, do therapy, teach, and write, it is totally unacceptable to me.

I, of course, have no way of knowing that my beliefs are true. However, for me, this is not as important as feeling intuitively—knowledge by being—that my story is right for me. Indeed, it helps me to accept, at least at one level, what has happened, even though at another level it is unlikely that my grief will ever end. What is more, the explorations that were involved in the process of creating my new story have changed me forever. In addition, I believe that as I have learned to live at two levels I have been able to expand my horizons far beyond what otherwise might have been the case.

Accordingly, living at two levels may mean opening up new parts of the self, or allowing new aspects of the self to emerge, in order to accommodate the loss and all that it entails. This may occur through a revised belief system, through choices to follow a path different from those previously chosen, through becoming a person who lives every day in the presence of grief and at the same time also is able to create a rich and full life. Indeed, as one changes in order to achieve stability, as one accepts a both/and perspective which acknowledges both sorrow and joy, one lives in awareness of the two levels that define the inevitable and basic paradoxes of life.

What is more, as professionals it is important to recognize that awareness of a transcendent dimension, of beliefs and values related to something larger than the self, is one of the processes characterizing successful families (Kaslow, 1982). It also has been identified as one of the essential components of family resilience (Walsh, 1998). And resilience is defined as the ability to meet and handle successfully both normal developmental challenges and unanticipated crisis and change. Thus, we may further support the healing process through recognition and support of attempts to live comfortably with both the material and the spiritual.

Encouraging laughter also may play an important role in this process, both facilitating an understanding of the two levels and enabling one's ability to live more comfortably and simultaneously in both. Humor is for me the "essential ingredient which warms and unites and makes the impossible possible—representative of as well as a solution to the paradoxes of existence" (Becvar, 1997, p. 16). In other words, "Whatever our hurt, there is a big difference between pain and suffering. Our pain may not cease, but humor can minimize our suffering by giving us power in what appears to be a powerless situation" (Allen, 1989, p. xx).

Humor offers relief, comic relief, in otherwise tragic circumstances, easing not only the mind but also often the body. In addition, humor provides a different perspective with which to view whatever problems or challenges may be faced. At first, those who are bereaved may feel unable to laugh or guilty if they do. Or laughter may quickly turn to tears. However, as they begin to laugh again they may recognize both that healing already has taken place and that they also are being healed by their laughter

Although humor will not take away our grief, it may enable us to cope more effectively with it. And when we can learn to laugh rather than cry at the ridiculous and potentially distressing situations that tend to try our patience, particularly when we are under stress, we may do ourselves an enormous favor. For, "In laughter, we transcend our predicaments. We are lifted above our feelings of fear, discouragement, and despair. People who can laugh at their setbacks no longer feel sorry for themselves. They feel uplifted, encouraged, and empowered" (Allen, 1989, p. 4). Given that there are likely to be many setbacks on the road to healing, it therefore may be important to invite those who are bereaved both to see the silliness in so much of what also is aggravating and give themselves permission to laugh as well as to cry.

One of the areas in which humor may be particularly helpful is in the challenging process of rebuilding life in the context of new meaning systems. Perhaps we may be able to encourage greater tolerance if we can laugh at ourselves and others and take our foibles and idiosyncracies a little less seriously. We may find that others have difficulty understanding or accepting the person we have become. First, they simply may not have a frame of reference for understanding our experience in anything but a superficial manner. We know well the world in which they live but they cannot possibly understand the dual reality—of the dead as well as the living—that we now inhabit. Second, as we are different with others, they may not know how to be with us. We may be violating the rules of our relationship and thus the relationship may no longer be viable. Third, others may feel uncomfortable with our changed views and behaviors. What we believe and the choices we make may be threatening or intimidating to others.

Once again, however, awareness of, as well as the ability to live at, two levels may assist us as we continue on our chosen paths. For as we can achieve an awareness that, at least at some larger level, there is something appropriate about whatever is occurring, we may be able to be more accepting of others in our world. What is more, it is highly likely that we will experience a change in priorities following the death of a loved one. Accordingly, it may become much more important to remain true to ourselves than to attempt to placate or please others, and we therefore also may be better able to accept the ending of relationships as they occur. Indeed, a greater sense of acceptance as well as a strong commitment to revised priorities may be just some of the many gifts offered to us by the experience of grief.

THE GIFTS OF GRIEF

How odd to think that grief brings gifts. However, not only is this case but such gifts are an extremely important contributor to and component of the ability of the bereaved to reclaim joy. Indeed, in the words of one who has worked intensively in the area of death and dying:

You may even come to feel mysteriously grateful toward your suffering, because it gives you such an opportunity of working through it and transforming it. Without it you would never have been able to discover that hidden in the nature and depths of suffering is a treasure of bliss. The times when you are suffering can be those when you are most open, and where you are extremely vulnerable can be where your greatest strength really lies. (Sogyal, 1992, p. 316)

For example, when someone loses a fear of death, which so often occurs following the loss of a loved one, he or she thereafter may experience life very differently. Most of all he or she may feel a great sense of freedom, or of liberation. For there is no more need for denial and one now can speak unselfconsciously and perhaps without any underlying anxiety about the inevitable. Indeed, the fact that a family member has already made the transition, perhaps coupled with a sense that she or he is just fine, may enable survivors to be confident that they, too, will be fine. It also may be reassuring to think that a beloved deceased person may be there waiting to greet the survivors when their time to die also comes.

Another important gift may be the ability to sort out and focus on that which really is most important and to let go of those things that are not. It therefore may be easier to take what look like risks at the level of physical reality in order to pursue and remain consistent with goals and values that emerge from awareness of the nonphysical level of existence. In other words, if integrity to the self and to one's principles becomes an overarching concern, the choice to leave situations, both personal and professional, in which a violation of these principles is experienced may be quite effortless. Although others may not understand such choices, they nevertheless may be appropriate, and thus not at all risky, given one's shifts in priorities.

Indeed, we may become much more aware of the need to nurture ourselves mentally and emotionally, as well as physically. We also may be much more willing to attend to needs in these areas. For as we come to terms with grief, life is likely to take on a new preciousness. We may be much more unwilling to sacrifice whatever time we may have out of respect both for ourselves and for the one who has died. We may even feel a sense of living for the one who has died and thus a greater feeling of mission and purpose about how this is done. We may understand each moment as valuable and we may consider only those encounters that do justice to this value as acceptable and therefore worthy of our time and energy.

At the same time, we also may find a greater acceptance of the views and choices of others despite their divergence from our own. Certainly we may be sad when we see people seemingly squandering their lives or not making the most of their talents. But we also may be much less judgmental. For who are we to say how anyone else should live when we ourselves have learned that there are no guarantees, that there are no solid answers for some of life's biggest questions? How can we attempt to control anyone else when we recognize how important it is to be able to live and act as we choose?

We also may be more accepting of life's small irritations and daily annoyances. There is no doubt that these will occur, that things will not always go as smoothly as we would like. We *will* get stuck in traffic; somebody *will* break a dish or spill milk; we *will* lose our keys and be late for an important appointment. However, we probably will find ourselves saying something like "Oh, well," or "that's a shame," in response and we will be less likely to become as totally bent out of shape as formerly might have been the case in such instances. Indeed, how can we allow ourselves to get so upset about such trivial things when we have experienced something so momentous?

Along with acceptance also may come the gift of compassion, not only for ourselves but also for those around us. Indeed, having experienced so much sorrow we may be able to feel much more deeply the pain of others. We may be much more willing to reach out to people who are in need. We may be much more able to sit with those who are grieving and just be present to whatever they may be feeling without a need to try to fix or change things for them. What is more, we will know that this is something we cannot do. And certainly we will have a much better idea about what may or not be helpful for them.

We probably will not offer platitudes. On the other hand, it is highly likely that we will call. We also may bring a gift of food. We will know to err on the side of intruding rather than hanging back. We also will send cards and letters, knowing how meaningful they can be, not only in the early days but also weeks and months later. As one bereaved mother learned and subsequently strongly urges:

> If a friend of yours loses someone, write them a letter full of love. You need them, these letters, to help get you through the days and evenings somehow. You open them, you read, you search through them for the *mot juste*, and you always find it. However distant the author of the letter may be, he is there,

vigilant; he helps you to look at your life; he says that he knows, that he is thinking, that he will keep and protect. The letters cement the bricks laid down by the survivors, Write, write, write. Do not miss one opportunity to do it. If you have the choice between writing and not writing, always choose to write. Not a single letter is out of place. We had letters from people who had heard us mentioned by mutual friends, people we had never met. Everything is a help. Each of us can be of help to everyone else. (Jurgensen, 1999, pp. 45–46)

One of the great gifts of grief is this knowing that may come regarding the experiences of others in our world. We will have walked the 10 miles in the moccasins they are now wearing. And somehow we may find that our hard edges have been softened in the process of being buffeted and tumbled by some of life's hardest challenges as we made our walk along the path of sorrow. Thus we may emerge feeling a deeper commitment to be of service, to facilitate healing for others, whether in large or small ways. We even may feel a sense of mission about letting others know that their journey also can have a joyful outcome.

And perhaps the greatest gift of all comes as we are able to reclaim joy. For, to our amazement, we may find that the ability to experience joy, as well as a recommitment to life and living as fully as possible, is exactly proportional to the degree of sorrow we also have known. Thus we may be much more responsive to the sights and sounds of our world. Music may be particularly meaningful, its beauty resonating at the deepest levels of our being. Similarly, a reality that had gone black and white now may be seen and appreciated in full technicolor. We may even come to respond with greater awareness and sensitivity to small moments of delight—kind words, a thoughtful gesture, a cloudless day. We also may feel an enhanced sense of both realism and idealism.

We know from firsthand experience that life can be very painful. We know that tragedies occur and that we may be part of them. But we also know that we have survived. We live in the presence of grief and yet we are able to be happy, at least for a portion of the time. Thus, not only may we be more appreciative of life's simple pleasures but also we may have a greater sense of what it is we can accomplish as well as a greater sense of satisfaction when we do so. We know what it means to be "joy-full."

Such ideas are for me expressed most eloquently in the following excerpt from *The Prophet*:

Then a woman said, Speak to us of Joy and Sorrow.
And he answered:
Your joy is your sorrow unmasked.
And the selfsame well from which your laughter rises was oftentimes
    filled with your tears.
And how else can it be?
The deeper that sorrow carves into your being, the more joy you can
    contain. (Gibran, 1923/1983, p. 28)

The final gift we must consider is that offered to professionals who have the opportunity, as well as the privilege, of working in the presence of grief. Many wonder why anyone would choose such an area of focus. They question whether or not it isn't morbid or depressing. And perhaps for them it might be. However, I have yet to meet someone who works either with those who are dying or with those who are bereaved who does not feel grateful to be able to help and support family members around end of life issues.

Being able to participate in the co-creation of new, more comfortable realities for clients in the context of death is a life-changing experience, one that also enhances and affirms the ability of helpers to appreciate life even as the death and dying experiences of others are improved. One need only envision the gradual shift in those who are bereaved from agonizing pain to the ability to reclaim a sense of joy to understand such sentiments.

We speak so easily and often about the miracle of life. If death is its logical complement, then must it not also be a miracle? Certainly I know a great deal about the pain as well as the joy associated with the former. I have given birth to and reared two children. I have assisted at the delivery of the child of a couple with whom I am very close. And I have welcomed the arrival and enjoyed both observing and nurturing the development of numerous other children, the sons and daughters of relatives, friends, and clients. I am deeply appreciative of the miracle of life.

Over the years, I also have learned a great deal about death. I have experienced the deaths of my son, both my parents, and many friends and relatives. As part of my role as a therapist I also have met and worked with numerous others who in a similar manner have been dealing with death, dying, bereavement, and related end-of-life issues. And I attempt each day to achieve greater understanding about and appreciation of the miracle of death, including the joy as well as the pain it also has the potential to create. I can honestly say that I feel a deep sense of gratitude for the experiences I have had in the arenas of both life and death. What is more, I feel that my world is enriched each day as I live and work in the presence of grief.

THERAPEUTIC CONVERSATIONS
AND REFLECTIONS

∽

I first met the Miller family in 1984. Kathleen and Bruce had three sons, Steven, Michael, and John. Although they had struggled for several years around Michael's sexual orientation, he recently had announced his certainty that he was gay and that he was no longer going to try to hide the fact. This was particularly devastating news given the family's religious belief system. Indeed, Kathleen and Bruce felt that they were being forced to make a choice between their church and their child. To complicate matters further, although Bruce was no longer active in this role, he was an ordained minister.

Although it was a decision with long-lasting ramifications, the family members were not willing to abandon their son and brother. Thus began a lengthy search for a new spiritual home. In addition, everyone had to learn to live with and accept Michael's homosexuality, a great challenge for them but one ultimately achieved.

Over the years various family members would come to therapy with me to work on a particular issue and then I would not hear anything for a while. I assisted with academic difficulties, career choices and changes, family-of-origin issues, and relationship problems. I also helped from time to time as the issue of Michael's homosexuality was revisited.

In the early 1990s, Michael learned that he was HIV+. He was able to enjoy a few more years of relatively good health. However, in December 1992, following some dental work, he contracted an infection and began having respiratory difficulties. He was hospitalized and following a bronchoscopy, was put on a ventilator. Kathleen, who was a trained nurse, immediately went to care for her son. He needed open-heart surgery, but at first the family was unable to find physicians willing to operate because of his HIV+ status.

(cont.)

When a team of surgeons finally was located, Michael was moved to another hospital and a lengthy and complicated operation was performed on Christmas eve.

By this time the entire family had arrived, having traveled from several different states to be with Michael and to support each other. The surgeon later remarked that he sometimes had found that the mothers came in such situations; that rarely did both parents come; and that never had he seen all the siblings be present as well. Fortunately, despite their worst fears and a poor prognosis, Michael survived the surgery. A month later Kathleen and Bruce brought him back to their home to recuperate.

I worked with Michael during this period of convalescence, going to his parents' home for weekly therapy sessions. Despite periodic nosebleeds, an after-effect of having been on the respirator, he was doing well. However, at the end of March 1993, he developed septicemia and died quickly. It was a terrible blow and followed within days a carjacking incident in which Bruce had nearly been beaten to death.

I recently met with Kathleen and asked her to describe how she had dealt with Michael's death in the early days. She said that she had surrounded herself with people who loved and supported her. She had gone back to work 2 weeks after Michael's death and had found the presence of caring colleagues to be very comforting. What is more, she felt that working had enabled her to ground herself, that otherwise she might just have "floated off." In the evenings, after work, she would play a tape of Michael's favorite music which the family had created for his memorial service and she would just wail until she was exhausted enough to be able to sleep.

In the years since Michael's death, Kathleen has continued to surround herself with people who are able to respect her need to tell her story. She also feels blessed that she had the opportunity to spend so much time with Michael before he died and that she has no regrets or guilt where he is concerned. Indeed, healing for all the family members occurred as they participated in caring for Michael at various times in his recovery process.

Today Kathleen feels very much at peace. She believes that her separation from Michael is not permanent, that when she dies he will be there waiting. She also has come to believe that the whole AIDS epidemic has a purpose. She feels that all the young men who have died from this disease are helping others in ways they could not do when they were alive. As for Michael, she trusts his journey, believing that he accomplished what he came to do and that he did not die before his time. She pictures him now counseling other souls and giving them comfort. She also feels him encouraging her and participating in her life, particularly when special songs come on the radio at significant moments in her life.

Kathleen attributes her ability to reclaim joy in her life to the presence of her then 3-year-old grandson and the subsequent birth of a second grandson. She found the small child's candor to be both delightful and comforting. He could ask questions and talk freely about his uncle. And the presence of both children continually reminds her of the ongoing cycle of life, death, and rebirth.

Today the family is able to have extremely enjoyable times together and they feel that tremendous growth has occurred for all of them. They continue to be loving and supportive. I believe their great love for one another has seen them through this great crisis and that they have come out in a wonderful place. It has been a joy to know and work with them.

The world loves closure, loves a thing that can, as they say, be gotten through. This is why it comes as a great surprise to find that loss is forever, that two decades after the event there are those occasions when something in you cries out at the continual presence of an absence.

—ANNA QUINDLEN

References

Achte, K. (1980). Death and ancient Finnish culture. In R. A. Kalish (Ed.), *Death and dying: Views from many cultures* (pp. 3–13). Farmingdale, NY: Baywood.

Allen, A. (1989). *The healing power of humor.* Los Angeles: Tarcher, Inc.

Allen, W. R. (1978). The search for applicable theories of black family life. *Journal of Marriage and the Family, 40*(4), 117–129.

American Association for Marriage and Family Therapy. (2001). *AAMFT code of ethics.* Washington, DC: Author.

Anderson, G., & Barone, A. (2000). *George Anderson's lessons from the light: Extraordinary messages of comfort and hope from the other side.* New York: Berkley Books.

Annas G. (1991). The health care proxy and the living will. *New England Journal of Medicine, 324*(17), 1210–1213.

Aries, P. (1962). *Centuries of childhood: A social history of family life.* New York: Vintage Books.

Aries, P. (1980). Forbidden death. In E. S. Shneidman (Ed.), *Death: Current perspectives* (2nd ed., pp. 52–55). Palo Alto, CA: Mayfield.

Baker, J. E. (1997). Minimizing the impact of parental grief on children: Parent and family interventions. In C. R. Figley, B. E. Bride, & N. Mazza (Eds.), *Death and trauma: The traumatology of grieving* (pp. 139–157). Washington, DC: Taylor & Francis.

Bank, S. P., & Kahn, M. D. (1982). *The sibling bond.* New York: Basic Books.

Barnhill, L., & Longo, D. (1978). Fixation and regression in the family life cycle. *Family Process, 17,* 469–478.

Bateson, G. (1972). *Steps to an ecology of mind.* New York: Ballantine Books.

Battin, M. (1994). *The least worse death.* New York: Oxford University Press.

Beauchamp T., & Childress J. (1994). *Principles of biomedical ethics* (4th Ed.). Oxford, England: Oxford University Press.

Becker, E. (1973). *The denial of death.* New York: Free Press.

Becvar, D. (1985). Creating rituals for a new age: Dealing positively with divorce, remarriage and other developmental challenges. In R. Williams, H. Lingren, G.

Rowe, S. Van Zandt, P. Lee, & N. Stinnett (Eds.), *Family strengths 6: Enhancement of interaction* (pp. 57–65). Lincoln: University of Nebraska–Lincoln.

Becvar, D. (1996, October). Assisted suicide: A spiritual perspective. *Family Therapy News*, p. 15.

Becvar, D. (1997). *Soul healing: A spiritual orientation in counseling and therapy.* New York: HarperCollins.

Becvar, D. (2000a). Euthanasia decisions. In F. W. Kaslow (Ed.), *Handbook of couple and family forensic issues* (pp. 439–458). New York: Wiley.

Becvar, D. (2000b). Families experiencing death, dying and bereavement. In W. C. Nichols, M. A., Nichols, D. S. Becvar, & A. Y. Napier (Eds.), *The handbook of family development and intervention* (pp. 453–470). New York: Wiley.

Becvar, D., & Becvar, R. (2000). *Family therapy: A systemic integration* (4th ed.). Boston: Allyn & Bacon.

Before the court, the sanctity of life and of death. (1997, January 5). *The New York Times*, p. 4E.

Berkus, R. (1984). *To heal again: Towards serenity and the resolution of grief.* Encino, CA: Red Rose Press.

Bernstein, J. (2000). *Bereft: A sister's story.* New York: North Point Press.

Bernstein, J. R. (1997). *When the bough breaks: Forever after the death of a son or daughter.* Kansas City, MO: Andrews & McKeel.

Billingsley, A. (1968). *Black families in white America.* Englewood Cliffs, NJ: Prentice-Hall.

Boss, P. (1991). Ambiguous loss. In F. Walsh & M. McGoldrick (Eds.), *Living beyond loss: Death in the family* (pp. 164–175). New York: Norton.

Boss, P. (1999). *Ambiguous loss: Learning to live with unresolved grief.* Cambridge, MA: Harvard Univesity Press.

Bouvard, M., & Gladu, E. (1998). *The path through grief: A compassionate guide.* New York: Prometheus Books.

Bowlby, J. (1980). *Loss, sadness and depression.* New York: Basic Books.

Bramblett, J. (1991). *When good-bye is forever: Learning to live again after the loss of a child.* New York: Ballantine Books.

Brodeur, D. (1997, August 31). Examining the American way of dying. *St. Louis Post Dispatch*, p. 3B.

Bronowski, J. (1978). *The origins of knowledge and imagination.* New Haven, CT: Yale University Press.

Brooks, J. (1999). *Midlife orphan: Facing life's changes now that your parents are gone.* New York: Berkley Books.

Brown, F. H. (1988). The impact of death on the family life cycle. In B. Carter & M. McGoldrick (Eds.), *The changing family life cycle: A framework for family therapy* (2nd ed., pp. 457–482). New York: Gardner Press.

Byng-Hall, J. (1991). Family scripts and loss. In F. Walsh & M. McGoldrick (Eds.), *Living beyond loss: Death in the family* (pp. 130–143). New York: W. W. Norton.

Byock, I. (1997). *Dying well.* New York: Riverhead Books.

Callahan, J. (1994). The ethics of assisted suicide. *Health and Social Work, 19*(4), 237–244.

Callahan, R. J., & Callahan, J. (1997). Thought field therapy: Aiding the bereavement process. In C. R. Figley, B. E. Bride, & N. Mazza (Eds.), *Death and trauma: The traumatology of grieving* (pp. 249–268). Washington, DC: Taylor & Francis.

Callanan, M., & Kelley, P. (1992). *Final gifts: Understanding the special awareness, needs, and communications of the dying.* New York: Bantam Books.

Carlson, L. (1987). *Caring for the dead: Your final act of love.* Hinesburg, VT: Upper Access.

Carter, S. L. (1996, July 21). Rush to a lethal judgment. *The New York Times Magazine,* pp. 28–29.

Carter, E. A., & McGoldrick, M. (Eds.), (1980). *The family life cycle: A framework for family therapy.* New York: Gardner Press.

Celocruz, M. T. (1992). Aid-in-dying: Should we decriminalize physician-assisted suicide and physician-committed euthanasia? *American Journal of Law and Medicine, 18*(4), 369–394.

Choice in Dying. (1991). *Refusal of treatment legislation—A state by state compilation of enacted and model statutes.* New York: Author.

Clay, R. (1997). Is assisted suicide ever a rational choice? *The APA Monitor, 28*(4), 1, 43.

Claypool, J. (1974). *Tracks of a fellow struggler: How to handle grief.* Waco, TX: Word Books.

Coddington, R. H. (1987). *Death brings many surprises.* New York: Ivy Books.

Conway, J. K. (1989). *The road from Coorain.* New York: Vintage Books.

Cousins, N. (1989). *Head first: The biology of hope.* New York: E. P. Dutton.

Daw, J. (1996, October). Assisted suicide: The facts. *Family Therapy News,* pp. 14, 28.

Deits, B. (1988). *Life after loss: A personal guide dealing with death, divorce, job change and relocation.* Tuscon, AZ: Fisher Books.

Demi, A., & Miles, M. (1987). Parameters of normal grief: A delphi study. *Death Studies, 11,* 397–412.

Doukas, D., & McCullough, L. (1991). The values history—The evaluation of the patient's values and advance directives. *Journal of Family Practice, 32*(2), 145–150.

Dreamer, O. M. (1999). *The invitation.* New York: HarperCollins.

Duvall, E. (1962). *Family development.* Philadelphia: Lippincott.

Dworkin, R. (1993). *Life's dominion—An argument about abortion and euthanasia.* London: Harper Collins.

Dworkin, J., & Kaufer, D. (1995). Social services and bereavement in the gay and lesbian community. In G. Lloyd & M. A. Kuszelewicz (Eds.), *HIV disease: Lesbians, gays and the social services* (pp. 41–60). New York: Harrington Press.

Dying Well Network. (1996). *Helping people die well.* Spokane, WA: Author.

Edelman, H. (1994). *Motherless daughters: The legacy of loss.* New York: Dell.

Eisdorfer, C., & Lawton, M. P. (Eds.), (1973). *The psychology of adult development and aging.* Washington, DC: American Psychological Association.

Erikson, E. (1963). *Childhood and society.* New York: Norton.

Farberman, R. K. (1997). *Terminal illness and hastened death requests: The important role of the mental health professional.* Washington, DC: American Psychological Association Press.

Feinstein, D. (1990). Cultivating and empowering mythology for confronting death. In D. Feinstein & P. E. Mayo, *Rituals for living and dying* (pp. 35–118). New York: HarperCollins.

Figley, C. R., Bride, B. E., & Mazza, N. (Eds.), (1997). *Death and trauma: The traumatology of grieving.* Washington, DC: Taylor & Francis.

Final Report of the Netherlands State Commission on Euthanasia: An English Summary (anonymous translation). (1987). *Bioethics, 1*(2), 163–174.

Fish, W. (1986). Differences of grief intensity in bereaved parents. In T. Rando (Ed.), *Parental loss of a child* (pp. 415–428). Champaign, IL: Research Press.

Foos-Graber, A. (1989). *Deathing: An intelligent alternative for the final moments of life.* York Beach, ME: Nicolas-Hays.

Freidman, E. H. (1980). Systems and ceremonies: A family view of rites of passage. In E. A. Carter & M. McGoldrick (Eds.), *The family life cycle: A framework for family therapy* (pp. 429–460). New York: Gardner Press.

Freud, S. (1957). Mourning and melancholia. In J. Strachey (Ed. and Trans.), *The standard edition of complete psychological works of Sigmund Freud* (Vol. 14, pp. 237–258). London: Hogarth Press and the Institute for Psychoanalysis. (Original work published 1917)

Fulton, R. (1987). The many faces of grief. *Death Studies, 11,* 243–256.

Gibran, K. (1983). *The prophet.* New York: Knopf. (Original work published 1923)

Gilbert, K. R. (1997). Couple coping with the death of a child. In C. R. Figley, B. E. Bride, & N. Mazza (Eds.), *Death and trauma: The traumatology of grieving* (pp. 101–121). Washington, DC: Taylor & Francis.

Gorer, G. (1980). The pornography of death. In E. S. Shneidman (Ed.), *Death: Current perspectives* (2nd ed., pp. 47–51). Palo Alto, CA: Mayfield.

Gottman, J. (1994). *Why marriages succeed or fail . . . and how you can make yours last.* New York: Simon & Schuster.

Gresham, D. H. (1988). *Lenten lands: My childhood with Joy Davidman and C. S. Lewis.* New York: HarperCollins.

Groopman, J. (1997). *The measure of our days: New beginnings at life's end.* New York: Viking.

Gunn, C. D. (1980). Family identity creation: A family strength-building role activity. In N. Stinnett, B. Chesser, J. DeFrain, & P. Knaub (Eds.), *Family strengths: Positive models for family life* (pp. 17–31). Lincoln: University of Nebraska Press.

Gutman, H. (1976). *The black family in slavery and freedom.* New York: Vintage Books.

Gutstein, S. E. (1991). Adolescent suicide: The loss of reconciliation. In F. Walsh & M. McGoldrick (Eds.), *Living beyond loss: Death in the family* (pp. 241–259). New York: Norton.

Hainer, C. (1997, August 11) At peace with death. *USA Today*, pp. 1–2D.

Hemlock Society. (1997, August). *Legislative matters.* pp. 1–6 [On-line]. Available: www.hemlock.org.

Hendin, H. (1995). *Suicide in America.* New York: Norton.

Hill, R. B. (1971). *The strengths of black families.* New York: Emerson Hall.

Hoffman, M. (1994). Use of advance directives: A social work perspective on the myth versus the reality. *Death Studies, 18,* 229–241.

Holmes, T. H., & Rahe, R. H. (1967). The social readjustment rating scale. *Journal of Psychosomatic Research, 11,* 213–218.

Hoopes, M. H., & Harper, J. M. (1987). *Birth order roles and sibling position in individual, marital, and family therapy.* Rockville, MD: Aspen.

Horwitz, S. H. (1997). Treating families with traumatic loss: Transitional family therapy. In C. R. Figley, B. E. Bride, & N. Mazza (Eds.), *Death and trauma: The traumatology of grieving* (pp. 211–230). Washington, DC: Taylor & Francis.

Houston, J. (1996). *A mythic life: Learning to live our greater story.* New York: HarperCollins.

Howard, G. S. (1991). Culture tales. *American Psychologist, 46,* 187–197.

Humphrey, D., & Clement, M. (2000). *People, politics and the right-to-die movement.* New York: St. Martin's Griffin.

Iglesias, T. (1995). Ethics, brain-death, and the medical concept of the human being. *Medical Legal Journal of Ireland,* pp. 51–57.

Imber-Black, E. (1991). Rituals and the healing process. In F. Walsh & M. McGoldrick (Eds.), *Living beyond loss: Death in the family* (pp. 207–223). New York: Norton.

Jackson, C. O. (1980). Death shall have no dominion: The passing of the world of the dead in America. In R. A. Kalish (Ed.), *Death and dying: Views from many cultures* (pp. 47–55). Farmingdale, NY: Baywood.

Jurgensen, G. (1999). *The disappearance.* New York: Norton.

Kalish, R. A. (Ed.). (1980). *Death and dying: Views from many cultures.* Farmingdale, NY: Baywood.

Kalish, R. A. (1985). The horse on the dining room table. In *Death, grief, and caring relationships* (2nd ed., pp. 2–4). Pacific Grove, CA: Brooks/Cole.

Kapleau, P. (1989). *The wheel of life and death.* New York: Doubleday.

Kaslow, F. (1982). Profile of the healthy family. *The Relationship, 8*(1), 9–25.

Kastenbaum, R. J. (1986). *Death, society, and human experience* (3rd. ed.). Columbus, OH: Charles E. Merrill.

Kelly, G. (1955). *The psychology of personal constructs.* New York: Norton.

Kennedy, A. (1991). *Losing a parent: Passage to a new way of living.* New York: HarperCollins.

Keown, D., & Keown, J. (1995). Killing, karma and caring: Euthanasia in Buddhism and Christianity. *Journal of Medical Ethics, 21,* 265-269.

Kielstein, R., & Sass, H. (1993). Using stories to assess values and establish medical directives. *Kennedy Institute of Ethics Journal, 3*(3), 303-325.

Kiser, J. D. (1996). Counselors and the legalization of physician-assisted suicide. *Counseling and Values, 40*(2), 127–131.

Klass, D. (1988). *Parental grief: Solace and resolution*. New York: Springer.

Klass, D., Silverman, P. R., & S. Nickman (Eds.), (1996). *Continuing bonds: New understandings of grief*. Washington, DC: Taylor & Francis.

Kleinman, A. (1988). *The illness narratives: Suffering, healing and the human condition*. New York: Basic Books.

Knapp, R. (1986). *Beyond endurance: When a child dies*. New York: Shocken.

Knapp, R. (1987, July). When a child dies. *Psychology Today*, pp. 60, 62–63, 66–67.

Kohner, N., & Henley, A. (1997). *When a baby dies: The experience of late miscarriage, stillbirth and neonatal death*. London: Thorsons.

Kreilkamp, A. (1999). Caring for our own dead: Interview with Jerri Lyons, founder and director The National Death Care Project. *Crone Chronicles, 41*, 20–30, 51.

Kübler-Ross, E. (1969). *On death and dying*. New York: Macmillan.

Kübler-Ross, E. (1975). *Death: The final stage of growth*. New York: Touchstone.

Kübler-Ross, E. (1995). *Death is of vital importance*. New York: Station Hill Press.

Kübler-Ross, E. (1997). *The wheel of life and death: A memoir of living and dying*. New York: Scribner.

Kushner, H. S. (1981). *When bad things happen to good people*. New York: Avon Books.

Ladner, J. A. (1973). Tomorrow's tomorrow: The black woman. In J. A. Ladner (Eds.), *The death of white sociology* (pp. 414–428). New York: Vintage Books.

LaFarge, P. (1982). The joy of family rituals. *Parents, 57*(12), 63–64.

Lambert, P., Gibson, J., & Nathanson, P. (1990). The values history: An innovation in surrogate medical decision-making. *Law, Medicine and Health Care, 18*(3), 202–212.

Lasch, C. (1979). *The culture of narcissism*. New York: Norton.

Lederer, W. J., & Jackson, D. D. (1968). *The mirages of marriage*. New York: Norton.

Lehman, D. R., Lang, E. L., Wortman, C. B., & Sorenson, S. B. (1989). Long-term effects of sudden bereavement: Marital and parent–child relationships and children's reactions. *Journal of Family Psychology, 2*, 344–367.

Levac, A. M. C., McLean, S., Wright, L. M., & Bell, J. M. (1998). A "reader's theater" intervention to managing grief: Posttherapy reflections by a family and clinical team. *Journal of Marital and Family Therapy, 24*(1), 81–93.

Levang, E. (1998). *When men grieve: Why men grieve differently and how you can help*. Minneapolis, MN: Fairview Press.

Levine, S. (1982). *Who dies? An investigation of conscious living and conscious dying*. New York: Doubleday.

Levine, S. (1997). *One year to live: How to live this year as if it were your last*. New York: Bell Tower.

Lewis, C. S. (1976). *A grief observed*. New York: Seabury Press.

Lewis, D. K. (1975). The black family: Socialization and sex roles. *Phylon*, XXXVI(3), 221–237.

Lightner, C., & Hathaway, N. (1990). *Giving sorrow words: How to cope with grief and get on with your life.* New York: Warner Books.

Lindbergh, A. M. (1998). *Dearly beloved.* New York: Buccaneer Books.

Lindemann, E. (1944). Symptomatology and management of acute grief. *American Journal of Psychiatry, 101,* 141–148.

Lopata, H. Z. (1996). Widowhood and husband sanctification. In In D. Klass, P. R. Silverman & S. L. Nickman (Eds.), *Continuing bonds: New understandings of grief* (pp. 149–162). Washington, DC: Taylor & Francis.

Lush, D. (1993). History of living wills. *Exchange on Aging Law and Ethics, 1*(2), 4–8.

Madden, K. (1999). *Shamanic guide to death and dying.* St. Paul, MN: Llewellyn.

Mair, M. (1988). Psychology as storytelling. *International Journal of Personal Construct Psychology, 1,* 125–138.

Martin, E. P., & Martin, J. M. (1978). *The black extended family.* Chicago: University of Chicago Press.

Martin, J., & Romanowski, P. (1994). *Our children forever: Messages from children on the other side.* New York: Berkley Books.

Mathis, A. (1978). Contrasting approaches to the study of black families. *Journal of Marriage and the Family, 40*(4), 667–676.

McAdoo, H. P. (1980). Black mothers and the extended family suppport network. In L. Rodgers-Rose (Ed.), *The black woman* (pp. 125–144). Beverly Hills, CA: Sage.

McClowry, S., Davies, E. B., May, K. A., Kulenkamp, E. J, & Martinson, I. M. (1987). The empty space phenomenon: The process of grief in the bereaved family. *Death Studies, 11,* 361–374.

McCracken, A., & Semel, M. (1998). *A broken heart still beats: After the death of a child.* Center City, MN: Hazelden.

McCrary, S., & Botkin, J. (1989). Hospital policy on advance directives: Do institutions ask patients about living wills? *Journal of the American Medical Association, 262*(17), 2411–2414.

McCullough, P., & Rutenberg, S. (1988). Launching children and moving on. In B. Carter & M. McGoldrick (Eds.), *The changing family life cycle: A framework for family therapy* (2nd ed., pp. 287–310). New York: Gardner Press.

McCutcheon, M. (1995). *Roget's super thesaurus.* Cincinnati: Writer's Digest Books.

McGoldrick, M., Almeida, R. Hines, P. M., Garcia-Preto, N., Rosen, E., & Lee, E. (1991). Mourning in different cultures. In F. Walsh & M. McGoldrick (Eds.), *Living beyond loss: Death in the family* (pp. 176–206). New York: Norton.

McGoldrick, M., & Walsh, F. (1991). A time to mourn: Death and the family life cycle. In F. Walsh & M. McGoldrick (Eds.), *Living beyond loss: Death in the family* (pp. 30–49). New York: Norton.

McLean, S. (1994, November 14). Paper presented at the International College of Surgeons, London.

McLean, S. (1996). End-of-life decisions and the law. *Journal of Medical Ethics, 22,* 261–262

Mehta, R. (1967). Introduction. In A. W. Osborn, *The expansion of awareness.* Wheaton, IL: Theosophical.

Mitford, J. (1963). *The American way of death.* New York: Simon & Schuster.

Mitford, J. (2000). *The American way of death revisited.* NY: Vintage Books.

Moody, R. A. (1977). *Life after life: The investigation of a phenomenon—survival of bodily death.* New York: Bantam Books.

Morse, M. (1990). *Closer to the light: Learning from the near-death experiences of children.* New York: Ivy Books.

Moss, M. S., & Moss, S. Z. (1996). Remarriage of widowed persons: A triadic relationship. In D. Klass, P. R. Silverman & S. L. Nickman (Eds.), *Continuing bonds: New understandings of grief* (pp. 163–178). Washington, DC: Taylor & Francis.

Nader, K. O. (1997a). Childhood traumatic loss: The interaction of trauma and grief. In C. R. Figley, B. E. Bride, & N. Mazza (Eds.), *Death and trauma: The traumatology of grieving* (pp. 17–41). Washington, DC: Taylor & Francis.

Nader, K. O. (1997b). Treating traumatic grief in systems. In C. R. Figley, B. E. Bride, & N. Mazza (Eds.), *Death and trauma: The traumatology of grieving* (pp. 159–192). Washington, DC: Taylor & Francis.

National Center for Health Statistics. (1996). Advance report of final mortality statistics (1994). *NCHS Monthly Vital Statistics Report, 45*(3, Suppl.).

Nickman, S. L., Silverman, P. R., & Normand, C. (1998). Children's construction of a deceased parent: The surviving parent's contribution. *American Journal of Orthopsychiatry, 68*(1), 126–134.

Nobles, W. W. (1978). Toward an empirical and theoretical framework for defining black families. *Journal of Marriage and the Family, 40*(4), 679–688.

Nolen-Hoeksema, S., & Larson, J. (1999). *Coping with loss.* Mahwah, NJ: Erlbaum.

Nouwen, H. J. M. (1994). *Our greatest gift: A meditation on dying and caring.* New York: HarperCollins.

Nurmi, L. A., & Williams, M. B. (1997). Death of a co-worker: Conceptual overview. In C. R. Figley, B. E. Bride, & N. Mazza (Eds.), *Death and trauma: The traumatology of grieving* (pp. 43–64). Washington, DC: Taylor & Francis.

O'Maley, C. (2000, February 24). Pet death should be taken seriously. *Butler Collegian* [On-line]. Available: www.butler.edu/dawgnet/000224/op-petdeath.html.

Osterweis, M., Solomon, F., & Green, M. (Eds.), (1984). *Bereavement: Reactions, consequences, and care.* Washington, DC: National Academy Press.

Otto, H. (1979). Developing human family potential. In N. Stinnett, B. Chesser, & J. Defrain (Eds.), *Building family strengths: Blueprints for action* (pp. 39–50). Lincoln: University of Nebraska Press.

Oxford dictionary of quotations. (1980). Oxford, England: Oxford University Press.

Packard, W. (Ed.). (1981). *Do not go gentle . . . : Poems on Death.* New York: St. Martin's Press.

Palmer, L. (1987). *Shrapnel in the heart: Letters and remembrances from the Vietnam Veterans Memorial.* New York: Random House.

Parkes, C. M., & Weiss, R. S. (1983). *Recovery from bereavement*. New York: Basic Books.

Peay, C. (1997, September–October). A good death. *Common Boundary*, pp. 32–41.

Peretz, D. (1970). Reaction to loss. In B. Schoenberg (Ed.), *Loss and grief* (pp. 20–35). New York: Columbia University Press.

Perrett, R. W. (1996). Buddhism, euthanasia and the sanctity of life. *Journal of Medical Ethics, 22,* 309–313.

Preston, T. A. (2000, May 22). Facing death on your own terms. *Newsweek*, p. 82.

Raheem, A. (1991). *Soul return: Integrating body, psyche and spirit*. Lower Lake, CA: Alan.

Rahimi, S. (1999). *Liberty to love legally (same-sex marriages)* [On-line]. Available: www.louisville.edu/a-s/english/wwwboard/neal/messages/88.html.

Rando, T. (1988). *Grieving: How to go on living when someone you love dies*. Lexington, MA: Lexington Books.

Rando, T. (1991). *How to go on living when someone you love dies*. New York: Bantam Books.

Rando, T. (1997). Foreword. In C. R. Figley, B. E. Bride, & N. Mazza (Eds.), *Death and trauma: The traumatology of grieving* (pp. xiv–xix). Washington, DC: Taylor & Francis.

Raphael, B. (1983). *The anatomy of bereavement*. New York: Basic Books.

Reif, L. V., Patton, M. J., & Gold, P. B. (1995). Bereavement, stress, and social support in members of a self-help group. *Journal of Community Psychology, 23,* 292–306.

Rigazio-DiGilio, S. A. (2001). Videography: Re-storying the lives of clients facing terminal illness. In R. Neimeyer, Ed., *Meaning reconstruction and the experience of loss* (pp. 331–344). Washington, DC: American Psychological Association.

Ring, K. (1984). *Heading toward omega: In search of the meaning of the near-death experience*. New York: William Morrow.

Roads, M. (1985). *Talking with nature*. Tiburon, CA: H. J. Kramer.

Rolland, J. (1991). Helping families with anticipatory loss. In F. Walsh & M. McGoldrick (Eds.), *Living beyond loss: Death in the family* (pp. 144–163). New York: Norton.

Rosen, H. (1986). *Unspoken grief: Coping with childhood sibling loss*. Lexington, MA: Lexington Books.

Rosenberg, M. A. (1986). *Companion animal loss and pet owner grief* [On-line]. The ALPO Pet Center. Available: www.berkshumane.org/memorial/petdeath.html.

Rothschild, J. (2000). *Signals: An inspiring story of life after life*. Novato, CA: New World Library.

Sarason, I. G., Sarason, B. G., Shearin, E. N., & Pierce, G. R. (1987). A brief measure of social support: Practical and theoretical implications. *Journal of Social and Personal Relationships, 4,* 497–510.

Sawin, M. M. (1979). *Family enrichment with family clusters*. Valley Forge, PA: Judson Press.

Sawin, M. M. (1982). *Hope for families*. New York: Sadlier.

Scanzoni, J. (1981, August). Family: Crisis or change? *The Christian Century*, pp. 794–799.

Scheper, T., & Duursma, S. (1994). Euthanasia: The Dutch experience. *Age and Aging, 23*, 3–8.

Schiff, H. S. (1977). *The bereaved parent*. New York: Penguin Books.

Sedney, M. A., Baker, J. E., & Gross, E. (1994). "The story" of a death: Therapeutic considerations with bereaved families. *Journal of Marital and Family Therapy, 20*(3), 287–296.

Shapiro, E. R. (1994). *Grief as a family process: A developmental approach to clinical practice*. New York: Guilford Press.

Sherman, H. (1981). *The dead are alive: They can and do communicate with you*. New York: Fawcett Gold Medal.

Shernoff, M. (1997). Individual practice with gay men. In G. Mallon (Ed.), *Foundations of social work practice*. New York: Harrington Park Press.

Shneidman, E. S. (Ed.). (1980a). *Death: Current perspectives* (2nd ed). Palo Alto, CA: Mayfield.

Shneidman, E. S. (1980b). Suicide. In E. S. Shneidman (Ed.), *Death: Current perspectives* (2nd ed., pp. 416–434). Palo Alto, CA: Mayfield.

Shneidman, E. S. (1996). *The suicidal mind*. New York: Oxford University Press.

Siegel, B. (1986). *Love, medicine and miracles*. New York: Harper & Row.

Silverman, P. R., & Klass, D. (1996). Introduction: What's the problem? In D. Klass, P. R. Silverman, & S. Nickman (Eds.), *Continuing bonds: New understandings of grief* (pp. 3–30). Washington, DC: Taylor & Francis.

Silverman, P. R., & Nickman, S. L. (1996). Concluding thoughts. In D. Klass, P. R. Silverman, & S. Nickman (Eds.), *Continuing bonds: New understandings of grief* (pp. 349–355). Washington, DC: Taylor & Francis.

Singlehood & Cohabitation (or "Nonmarital lifestyles" [On-line]). (2000). Available: www.clas.ufl.edu/users.kjoos.syg2430;singlelecture.htm.

Smith, H. I. (1996). *Grieving the death of a friend*. Minneapolis, MN: Augsburg Fortress.

Sogyal, R. (1992). *The Tibetan book of living and dying*. New York: HarperCollins.

Solomon, R. M., & Shapiro, F. (1997). Eye movement desensitization and reprocessing: A therapeutic tood for trauma and grief. In C. R. Figley, B. E. Bride, & N. Mazza (Eds.), *Death and trauma: The traumatology of grieving* (pp. 231–248). Washington, DC: Taylor & Francis.

Speckhard, A. (1997). Traumatic death in pregnancy: The significance of meaning and attachment. In C. R. Figley, B. E. Bride, & N. Mazza (Eds.), *Death and trauma: The traumatology of grieving* (pp. 101–121). Washington, DC: Taylor & Francis.

Starhawk, N. M. M., & The Reclaiming Collective. (1997). *The pagan book of living and dying*. New York: HarperCollins.

Steinberg, A. (1997). Death as a trauma for children: A relational treatment approach. In C. R. Figley, B. E. Bride, & N. Mazza (Eds.), *Death and trauma: The traumatology of grieving* (pp. 123–137). Washington, DC: Taylor & Francis.

Steiner, R. (1968). *Life between death and rebirth*. Spring Valley, NY: Anthroposophic Press.

Strommen, M. P., & Strommen, A. I. (1993). *Five cries of grief*. New York: HarperCollins.

Sulloway, F. J. (1996). *Born to rebel: Birth order, family dynamics, and creative lives*. New York: Pantheon Books.

Toman, W. (1961). *Family constellation*. New York: Springer.

Toynbee, A. (1980). Various ways in which human beings have sought to reconcile themselves to the fact of death. In E. S. Shneidman (Ed.), *Death: Current perspectives* (2nd ed., pp. 11–34). Palo Alto, CA: Mayfield.

Umberson, D., & Chen, M. D. (1994). Effects of a parent's death on adult children: Relationship salience and reaction to loss. *American Sociological Review, 59*, 152–168.

U.S. Public Health Service. (2000). *Suicide statistics*. Washington, DC: National Center for Health Statistics, Office of the Surgeon General.

VA Medical Center. (1993). *Advance directives—making decisions about your health care*. Seattle, WA: Author.

Van Auken, S. (1977). *A severe mercy*. San Francisco: Harper & Row.

Van Praagh, J. (2000). *Healing grief: Reclaiming life after any loss*. New York: Penguin Putnam.

Walsh, F. (1988). The family in later life. In B. Carter & M. McGoldrick (Eds.), *The changing family life cycle: A framework for family therapy* (2nd ed., pp. 311–332). New York: Gardner Press.

Walsh, F. (1998). *Strengthening family resilience*. New York: Guilford Press.

Warch, W. (1977). *The new thought Christian*. Marina del Rey, CA: DeVorss.

Watts, D. T. (1992). Assisted suicide is not voluntary active euthanasia. *Journal of the American Geriatrics Society, 40*(10), 1043–1046.

Watzlawick, P. (1978). *The language of change*. New York: Basic Books.

Weir, R. F. (1992). The morality of physician-assisted suicide. *Law, Medicine and Health Care, 20*(1–2), 116–126.

Whitton, J. L., & Fisher, J. (1986). *Life between life*. New York: Warner Books.

Williams, M. B., & Nurmi, L. A. (1997). Death of a co-worker: Facilitating the healing. In C. R. Figley, B. E. Bride, & N. Mazza (Eds.), *Death and trauma: The traumatology of grieving* (pp. 193–207). Washington, DC: Taylor & Francis.

Wolin, S. J., & Bennett, L. A. (1984). Family rituals. *Family Process, 12*(3), 401–420.

Wolterstorff, N. (1987). *Lament for a son*. Grand Rapids, MI: William B. Eerdmans.

Woods, R. I. (Ed.). (1957. *A treasury of friendships*. New York: David McKay.

Young, E., & Jex, S. (1992). The Patient Self-Determination Act: Potential ethical quandries and benefits. *Cambridge Quarterly of Healthcare Ethics, 2*, 107–115.

Zisook, S., & Shucter, S. (1986). The first four years of widowhood. *Psychiatric Annals, 16*(5), 288–294.

Zonnebelt-Smeenge, S. J., & De Vries, R. C. (1998). *Getting to the other side of grief: Overcoming the loss of a spouse*. Grand Rapids, MI: Baker Books.

Index